The Kock Pouch

Pär Myrelid • Mattias Block

Editors

The Kock Pouch

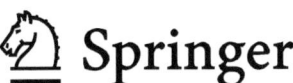 Springer

Editors
Pär Myrelid
Linköping University Hospital
Department of Surgery
Linköping University
Department of Clinical
and Experimental Medicine
Linköping, Sweden

Mattias Block
Department of Surgery
Colorectal Unit
Sahlgrenska University Hospital
Östra, Göteborg, Sweden

ISBN 978-3-319-95590-2   ISBN 978-3-319-95591-9   (eBook)
https://doi.org/10.1007/978-3-319-95591-9

Library of Congress Control Number: 2018961571

This Springer imprint is published by the registered company Springer Nature Switzerland AG
The registered company address is: Gewerbestrasse 11, 6330 Cham, Switzerland

Preface

The continent ileostomy, or the Kock pouch, is named after its inventor and creator, Professor Nils G. Kock (1924–2011). Professor Kock originated from Jakobstad, Finland, but spent most of his carrier working in Göteborg, Sweden, from the mid-1950s to 1990. He became professor in 1974. In 1969, he described the continent ileostomy as an alternative to the Brooke ileostomy after proctocolectomy for Ulcerative Colitis and Familial Polyposis.

The aim and rationale of the Kock pouch was the possibility for patients to have an option eliminating the necessity of an external ostomy appliance and to improve quality of life by providing continence for gas and feces. Patients were able to use normal clothing, swimsuits etc. and to experience a very good quality of life. Professor Kock early realized that education in basic research is an important platform for clinical and scientific activities and therefore started an animal study model supervised by Professor Björn Folkow in the Department of Physiology at the University of Göteborg before implementing the Kock pouch in the clinic.

The Kock pouch underwent several modifications and improvements during the first years, formation of the nipple in 1972 being one of the most important ones. By intussusception of the outlet segment, a nipple valve was constructed to improve the problem of leakage that many patients experienced earlier.

In 1977, stapling devices were introduced in abdominal surgery by Professor Félicien Steichen, and Professor Kock adapted this technique in stapling of the nipple by using four rows of staples to secure the nipple valve. Marlex mesh was used in the 1980s but was abandoned due to fistula formation. Since 1986, creation of the Kock pouch has more or less being unaltered.

Patients with a well-functioning Kock pouch are extremely satisfied and have a very good quality of life. However, creation of the Kock pouch is a complex procedure, and even in very experienced hands, the cumulative risk of reoperations appears to be about 45% at 15–20 years. The most common problems are leakage and intubation problems, usually due to slippage of the nipple.

Development of the ileal pouch-anal anastomosis (IPAA) in 1980, combined with the risk for reoperations, led to that many surgeons preferred to offer patients an IPAA instead of a Kock pouch in order to offer patients a life without a stoma.

However, all patients are not suited for an IPAA (perianal disease and anatomical variations being some factors), and for patients that really want to avoid a stoma, the Kock pouch still plays an important role. Another important fact is that there are many patients around the world that have a Kock pouch, and these patients can eventually end up with problems that need surgical care and in some cases surgical revision. So forth, the competence and knowledge of the pouch and how to perform revisional surgery as well as understand the Kock pouch and its consequences are very important knowledge to pass on to future surgeons and nursing staff taking care of patients with a Kock pouch.

Therefore, we believe that this book is an important contribution to the knowledge of the Kock pouch, the continent ileostomy, and we hope that patients with Kock pouch in the future can feel safe about having the optimal treatment and care of their Kock pouch, both by surgeons and nursing staff. This book covers the history and evolution of the Kock pouch, the different techniques used, indications and contraindications, pre- and postoperative care, follow-up, complications, pouchitis, revisional surgery, failure, and much more.

We believe that this book can be of great use in the clinic by health-care personnel that provides care for patients with a Kock pouch and also as a reference tool and encyclopedia for health-care personnel in general.

We wish you all a good reading!

Gothenburg, Sweden   Mattias Block
Linköping, Sweden   Pär Myrelid

Contents

Chapter 1
History of the Continent Ileostomy

Helge E. Myrvold and Leif Hultén

In 1969 Nils G. Kock described the continent ileostomy as an alternative to the Brooke ileostomy after proctocolectomy for Ulcerative Colitis and Familial Polyposis, the aim and rational being to eliminate the necessity of an external ostomy appliance and to improve quality of life in the patients by providing continence for gas and feces.

The theoretical considerations and experimental studies leading to the principle of the continent ileostomy emanated from the early 60s when Kock worked in the Department of Urology at Sahlgrenska University Hospital in Göteborg, Sweden. At that time, intestinal segments were widely used as bladder substitutes after total or partial cystectomy. Either an ileal or a colonic segment was sutured to the trigonum or urethra [1–4]. However, the functional results were less satisfying due to incontinence, especially at night.

At an early stage of his career, Kock realized that education in basic research is an important platform for clinical and scientific activities and therefore started an animal-study supervised by professor Björn Folkow at the Department of Physiology at the University of Göteborg. He published his thesis" An experimental analysis of mechanisms engaged in reflex inhibition of intestinal motility'" and received his PhD in 1959 [5]. To elucidate the problems of the bladder substitutes, he established subsequently a laboratory for urodynamic studies at the Department of Surgery and adapted the recording device for pressure studies on the bladder substitutes. Studying the pressure characteristics during graded filling of the substitutes he

H. E. Myrvold (✉)
Department of Clinical and Molecular Medicine, NTNU – Norwegian University of Science and Technology, Trondheim, Norway
e-mail: helge.myrvold@ntnu.no

L. Hultén
Department of Surgery Colorectal Unit, Sahlgrenska University Hospital SU/Ö, Göteborg, Sweden
e-mail: leif.hulten@surgery.gu.se

© Springer Nature Switzerland AG 2019
P. Myrelid, M. Block (eds.), *The Kock Pouch*,
https://doi.org/10.1007/978-3-319-95591-9_1

noted that strong pressure waves were generated already at low volumes - both in the ileal and sigmoid substitutes - pressure waves that exceeded the resistance of the urethral sphincter and caused leakage (Figs. 1.1 and 1.2).

In 1953, Tasker TH – urologist at Sheffield Royal Hospital – had reported on a new promising "detubularizing" technique to increase the capacity of the neobladder by splitting the isolated intestinal loop along its antimesenteric border, folding it into a U and closing it by suturing it side-to-side. Cystometrogram of this bladder design did

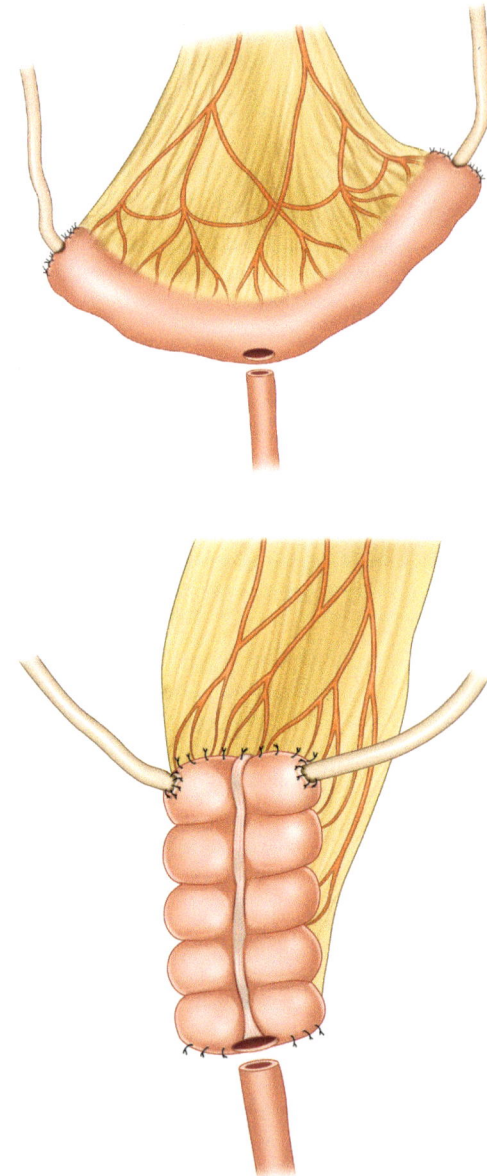

Fig. 1.1 Urinary bladder substitute formed by a tubular ileum segment. Flow cystometry have shown that already after infusion of 100 ml the pressure exceeds the urinary sphincter resistance and leakage occur

Fig. 1.2 Sigmoid bladder substitute. After infusion of 150 ml bladder pressure waves above 100 cm H_2O occurred and leakage via urethra occurred

not generate high-pressure waves until higher-filling volumes (Fig. 1.3). Kock was inspired by these results and suggested another folding technique. After splitting the intestinal loop - instead of folding it side-to-side - the ileal segment was folded top-down – making it a spherical configuration (Fig. 1.4). Cystometrogram demonstrated a minor increase in basal pressure and only a few low-pressure waves appeared on slow infusion of fluid into the reservoir (Fig. 1.4). This pouch design was subsequently used as an orthotopic bladder substitute in a number of patients and proved to yield a large volume capacity with a satisfactory function [6]. Yet the method never gained the popularity it actually deserved and fell into disuse for unclear reasons.

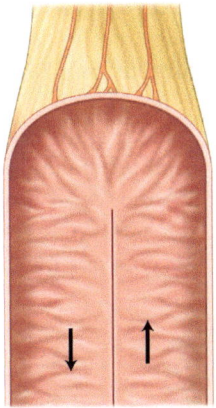 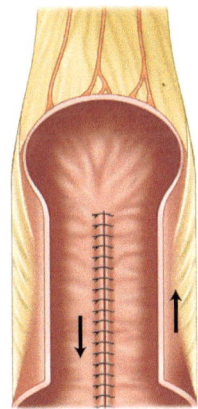 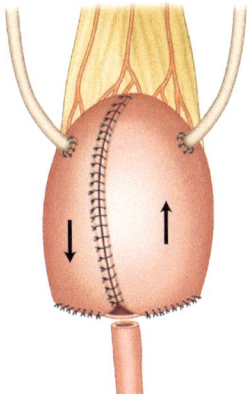

Fig. 1.3 Tasker bladder. Pressure studies (cystometry) demonstrated only a slight increase in basal pressure. Up to 200 ml infused pressure waves above 75 cm H_2O did not occur

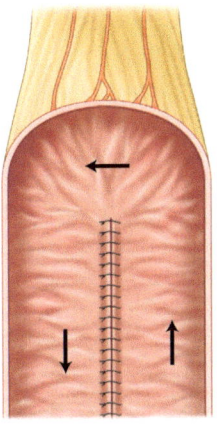 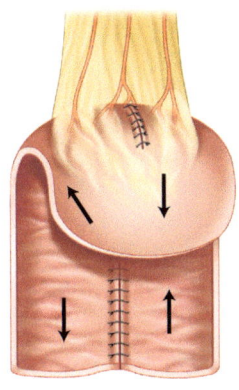 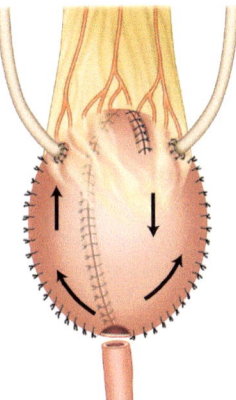

Fig. 1.4 Bladder substitute according to Kock's "double folded" technique. Pressure studies (cystometry) demonstrated only a slight increase in basal pressure and no pressure waves occurred at 350 ml infused

1.1   Creation of the Continent Ileostomy

Kock realized that this type of low-pressure reservoir also should be appropriate for collection and storage of intestinal discharge and started a clinical study – using the" low-pressure reservoir" as a continent ileostomy in patients after proctocolectomy. The reservoir was constructed from distal ileum (Fig. 1.5). In the first patients, a" corner" of the reservoir was simply passed through the rectus muscle and sewn to the skin with a mucocutaneous suture as done in a conventional stoma. It was thought that the rectus muscles might compress the pouch stoma and prevent leakage. A preliminary report was published in 1969 [7]. The volume of the reservoir – 50 ml at construction increased gradually during a few weeks to about 600 ml, which proved to be a convenient capacity allowing for evacuation of the reservoir by catheter about three to four times daily. Although some patients managed fairly well using only a small piece of gas covering the stoma, most patients experienced leakage, especially at straining and coughing and therefore patients had to use an external appliance. In attempts to improve continence Kock provided the reservoir either with anti-peristaltic- (Fig. 1.6) or isoperistaltic outlet (Fig. 1.7) in the next series of patients [8] but the results were inconsistent. Therefore, the concept of the nipple valve was introduced (Fig. 1.8).

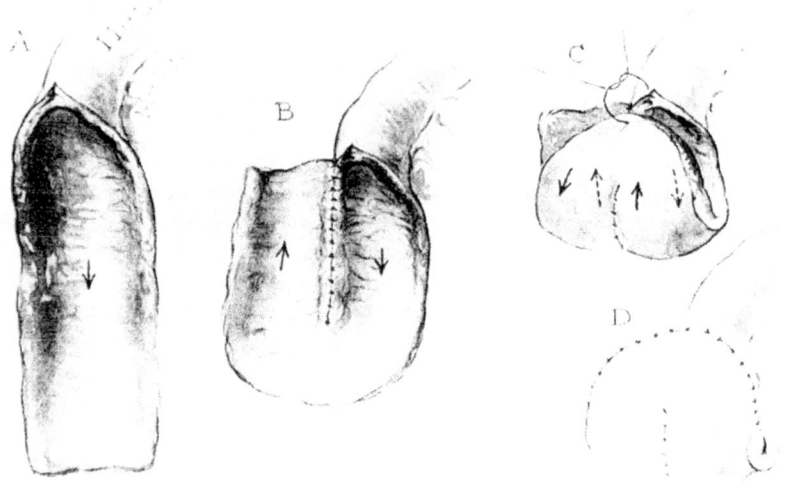

Fig. 1.5 Kock's original construction of the ileostomy reservoir. A corner of the reservoir was passed through the rectus abdominis musculature and sewn to the skin as a flat Ileostomy. Five patients were provided with this type of reservoir

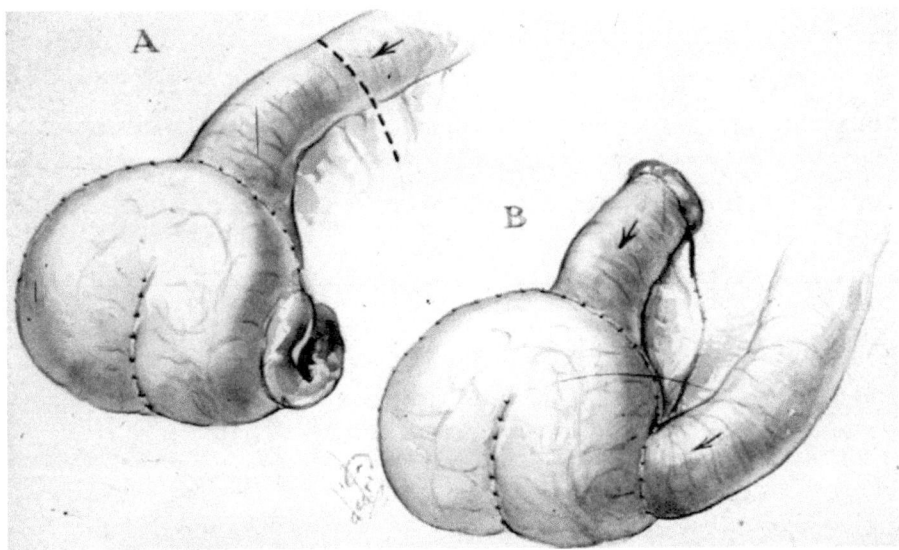

Fig. 1.6 Construction of reservoir with antiperstaltic outlet. This method was used in 35 patients

1.1.1 The Nipple Valve

A further important step in the evolution of the technique was taken 1972. By intussusception of the outlet segment, a nipple valve was constructed (Fig. 1.9) [9]. Although most patients were continent initially others experienced leakage of gas and faeces within the passage of time. Fistula formation at the site of the suturing of the nipple valve proved sometimes to be the explanation. However, more often incontinence was caused by desusception of the nipple valve - a "slippage" occurring mainly along the mesenteric part of the valve (Fig. 1.10). The bulk of the mesentery was supposed to prevent firm fixation and on reservoir expansion the two layers of the nipple valve tended to tear apart [8].

Different methods, such as application of a special "rotation suture", serosal scarification, reinforcing the nipple valve with a fascia slingtransplant and/or a marlex mesh were tried, but failed to overcome the problem of nipple valve slippage. Serosal stripping and defattening of the mesentery seemed to be beneficial and have remained as important parts of the nipple valve contruction (Fig. 1.11).

In 1977, professor Felicien Steichen introduced stapling in abdominal surgery [10]. Kock adapted this technique and in following experimental studies in dogs established the usefulness of stapling the nipple valve. Kock used four rows of staples to secure the nipple valve (Fig. 1.12) and a marlex mesh around the nipple base. This method was used from 1978 to the early 80s. The use of fascia sling and marlex mesh was hampered

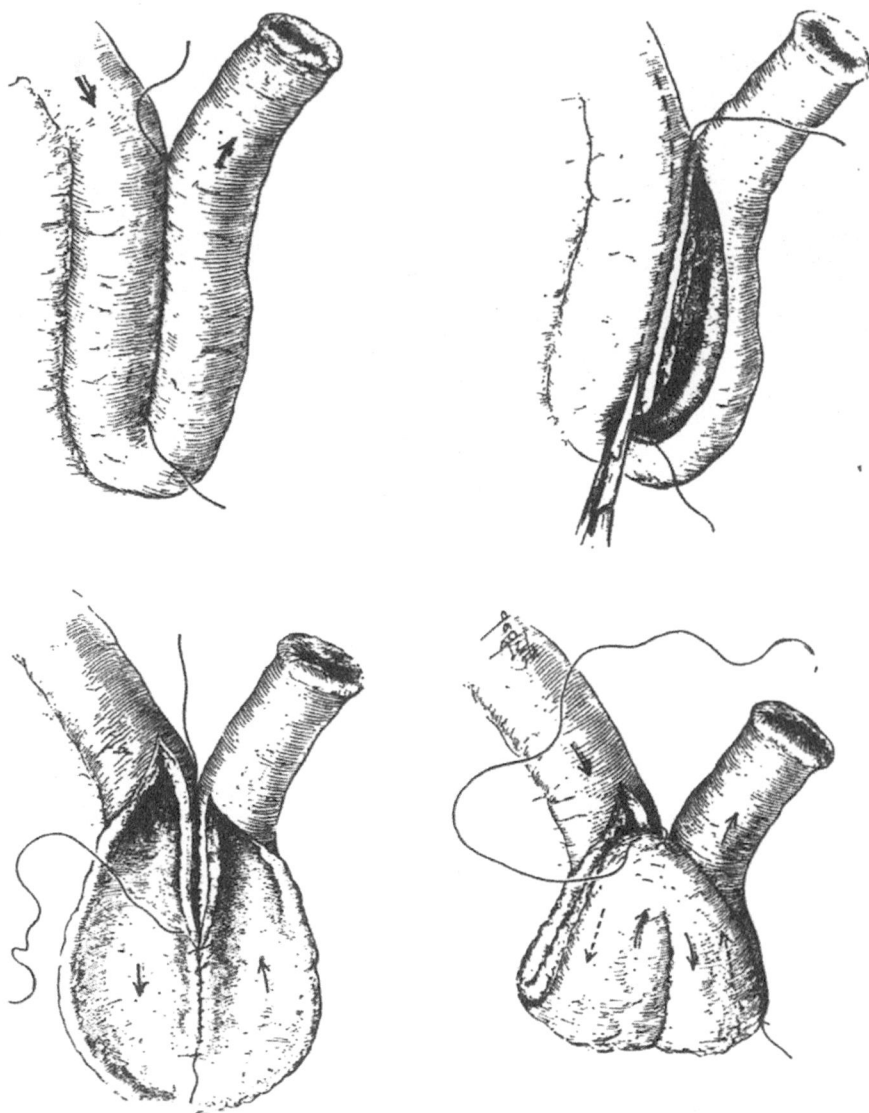

Fig. 1.7 Construction of reservoir with isoperistaltic outlet. This method was used in 31 patients

by fistula formation and thus omitted in the next and final version published in 1986 [11]. To further secure the nipple valve, it was anchored by one of the staple rows to the reservoir wall (Fig. 1.13). Thus, in the final and present version of the nipple valve it is constructed by invagination of the isoperistaltic outlet and secured with four rows of staples, one of them including the reservoir wall. This last staple row secure and prevent sliding of the nipple valve [11]. Prolonged postoperative intubation of the reservoir to stabilize the nipple valve was an important measure as suggested by Gelernt [12].

Fig. 1.8 Continent
ileostomy in situ

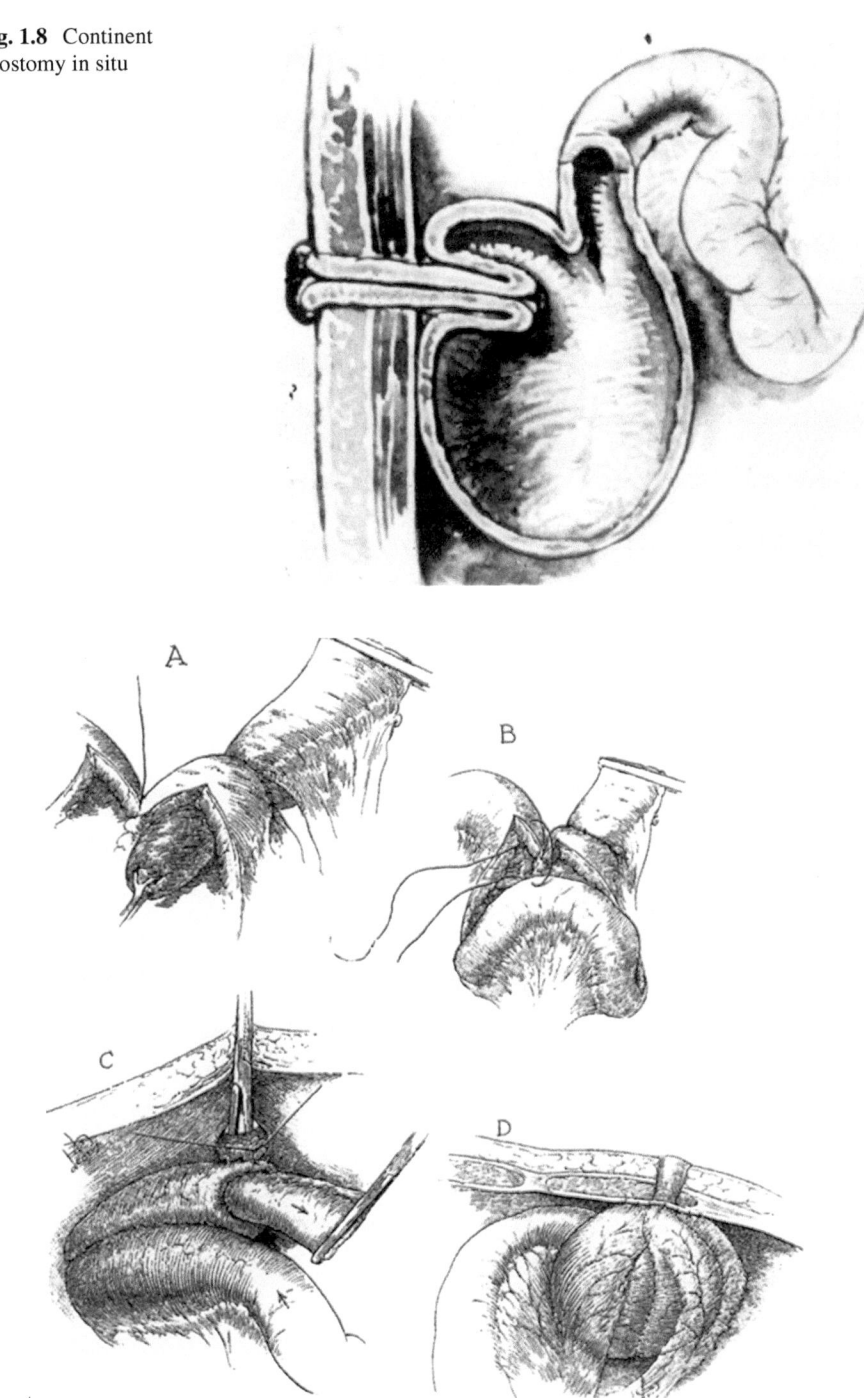

Fig. 1.9 Construction of ileostomy reservoir with nipple valve created by intususception of the
outlet into the reservoir

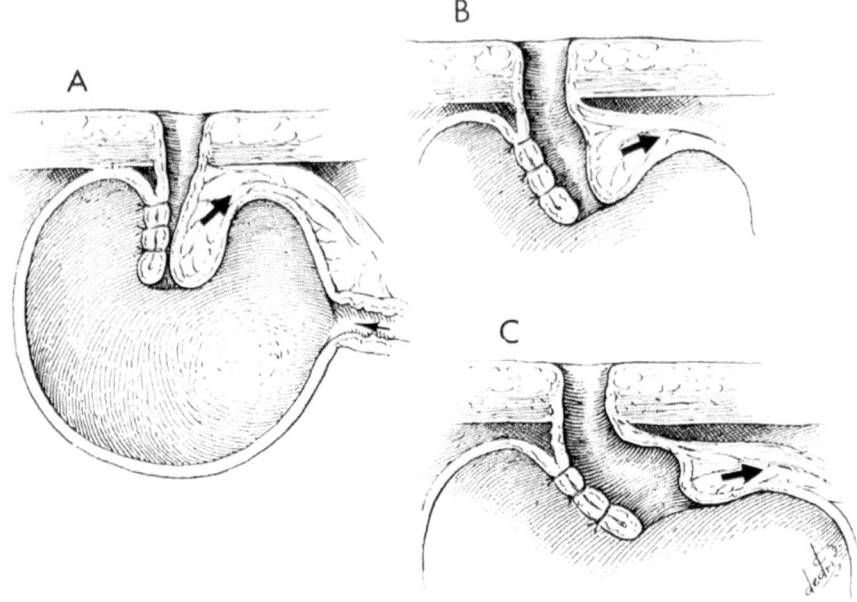

Fig. 1.10 Mechanism of nipple valve sliding

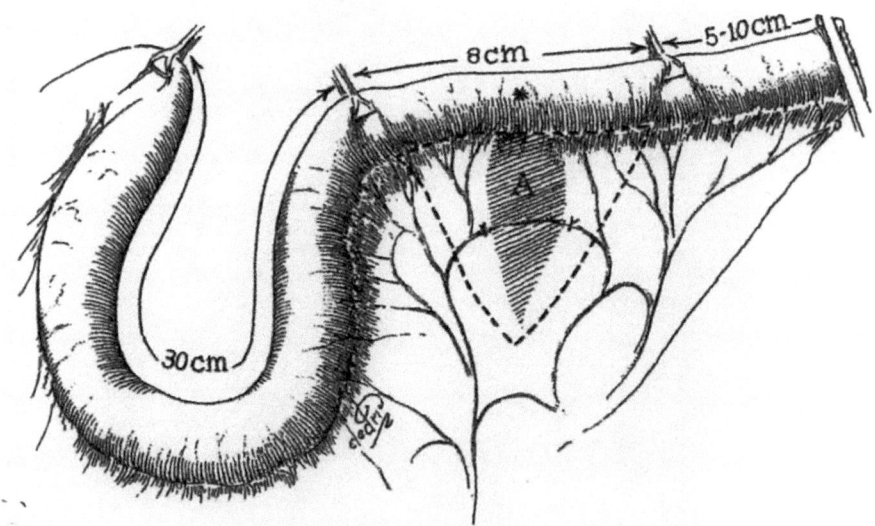

Fig. 1.11 Triangular stripping of the peritoneum and defattening of mesentery

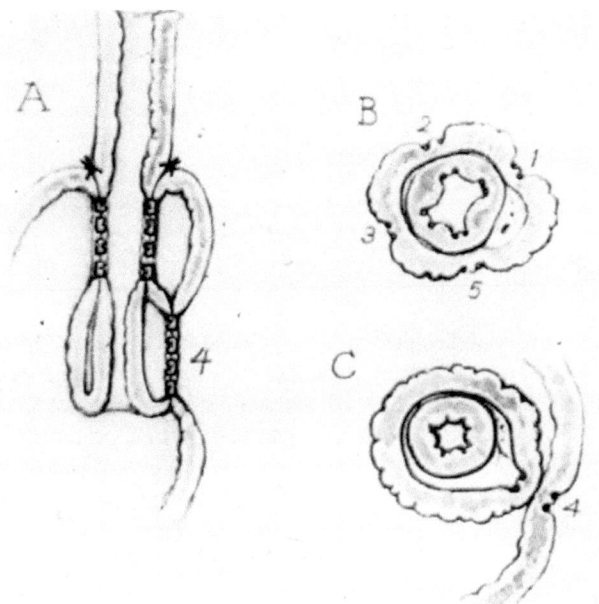

Fig. 1.12 The nipple valve constructed by invagination of the isoperistaltic outlet secured with four rows of staples, one of them including the reservoir wall

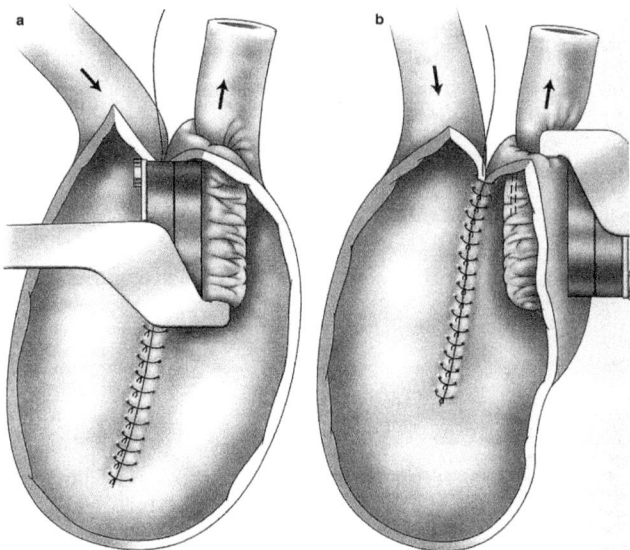

Fig. 1.13 Stapling the nipple valve. The nipple valve is anchored to the reservoir wall by one of the staple rows. (Reprinted by permission of Springer. Complexities in Colorectal Surgery by Scott R. Steele, Justin A. Maykel, Bradley J. Champagne, Guy R. Orangio. Editors)

Barnett modified the method using the afferent loop for outlet and an intestinal segment wrapped around the outlet [13, 14]. Kaiser and Beart developed the T-pouch replacing the nipple valve with an isolated ileal segment [15, 16]. Although good results were presented, the methods are complicated and have not reached wide acceptance among the surgical society.

1.2 Physiological Consequences and Biological Consequences

Extensive physiological studies during the 70ies and early 80ies revealed that the volume and motility patterns are closely related to the length of the postoperative observation time, indicating an adaption of the reservoir smooth muscles to distention The pouch volume increases rapidly from less than 100 ml to approximately 600 ml after 6 months and then remain stable (Fig. 1.14). Pressure waves and motor activity decrease to almost negligible measures during the first year after surgery [17–19]. Pressure studies of the nipple valve confirmed its ability to maintain continence [20–22].

It has been argued that the continent ileostomy might develop a stagnant loop syndrome with passage of time. B12 malabsorption, increased bile acid excretion and steatorrhea have been reported [23–26]. The physiological and biologic consequences have been studied extensively primarily in Sweden but also worldwide. It is clear that the bacterial flora of the pouch takes an intermediate position between the terminal ileum and faeces, both in quality and quantity [27]. Morphological changes include broadening and decrease in the height of the villi as well as increase of the number of mitosis in the crypt cells [28]. None of these changes appear to be harmful in long term follow-up studies over 10–18 years [29, 30]. There was no evidence of vitamin B12 malabsorption caused by the ileal pouch [31]. Furthermore, it has been shown that vitamin B12 is

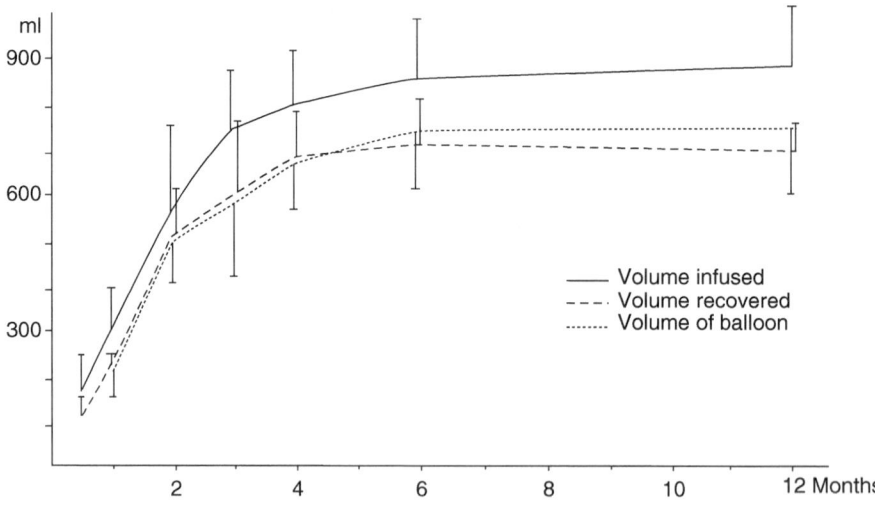

Fig. 1.14 The volume capacity with the passage of time after construction

absorbed from the pouch [19]. The majority of patients exhibits normal B12 levels with no need for general subsitution. There is an increased loss of bile acids, but this is not reflected in fat malabsorption [29]. The patients adapt very well to the loss of colon and show no signs of water or electrolyte depletion in long term follow up [32–35]. The physiological and biological studies of the continent ileostomy do not disclose adverse events and confirms the safety of the continent ileostomy in clinical praxis. However, given that a lifetime with an ileal pouch is to be expected, the occurrence of even border-line malabsorption should not be ignored.

1.3 Clinical Results

The great majority of patients provided with a continent ileostomy at Sahlgrenska University Hospital, Göteborg, Sweden were operated for Ulcerative Colitis or Familial Polyposis, but also included a number of patients with Crohn's disease[9, 36–40].

The construction of the continent ileostomy has been afflicted with a relatively high incidence of immediate and late complications, most of them have been related to the nipple valve; fistulas related to the through and through sutures, use of foreign material for stabilization and desusception of the valve by sliding on the mesenteric side as depicted in Fig. 1.10. Due to the increased surgical experience and by applying the sta-pling technique for the nipple valve, the occurrence of complications have decreased considerably. Both operative mortality and non-fatal complications decreased consider-ably from 4.3% mortality and 23% nonfatal complications during 1967–1974 to 0% and 8% respectively during 1975–1984 [11, 37, 40, 41]. Similar results and decrease in complication rates have been reported from various institutions worldwide [41–50]. Cumulative rates of reoperation appears to be about 45% at 15–20 years [30, 49]. The most common complication is inflammation of the pouch ileal mucosa (pouchitis). Occurrence of pouchitis varies considerably, possibly due to variable definitions, but usually ends up at around 30% of patients having episodes with pouchitis [44, 45, 49, 51]. Pouchitis is in most cases effectively treated medically. Despite complication rates and the need for reoperations, all published studies confirm the great satisfaction of the patients as reported in several quality of life studies.

It is a general agreement that patients operated for Ulcerative Colitis or Familial Polyposis are those most suitable for the continent ileostomy. Patients with Crohn's disease are usually considered not eligible for the procedure although success have been reported in highly selected patients with Crohn's disease.

It is notable that by creating an ileal reservoir for collecting faeces, Kock actually pawed the way for the ileal pouch-anal anastomosis. Sir Alan Parks at St. Marks Hospital in London applied the principle of the continent ileostomy reservoir, but constructed the reservoir using three loops folded as an S instead of the double fold-ing of the Kock pouch. He moved the reservoir to the pelvis and the outlet to the anus preserving the anal sphincter thus creating an ileal pouch-anal anastomosis. He published the method in 1978 [52, 53]. Initially the patients had problems with emptying because of the long outlet and 50% of the patients had to empty the reser-voir by perianal intubation. Interestingly, in 1968 Kock anastomosed the pouch to a patient's anal sphincter via a five cm long ileal outlet. The patient was continent but had to empty the pouch with a catheter introduced via anus. Due to the inconvenience of the emptying procedure and irritation of the anus, the pelvic pouch was converted to a continent ileostomy. Later (1989) Kock introduced the Kock pouch for ileal pouch-anal anastomosis as described in Chap. 7 [54].

1.4   Continent Urostomy and Orthotopic Bladder Substitute

In the early 1970s, Kock explored the possibility of using the ileal reservoir for continent urostomy. After a series of experiments in dogs [55] the first patient was operated in 1975 at the Department of Urology at Sahlgrenska University Hospital. In 1982, the results of 12 patients was published [56] and in 2002 long-term follow up of 176 patients were reported [57]. The continent urostomy is provided with a second nipple to prevent reflux (Fig. 1.15) [58]. The Kock continent urostomy

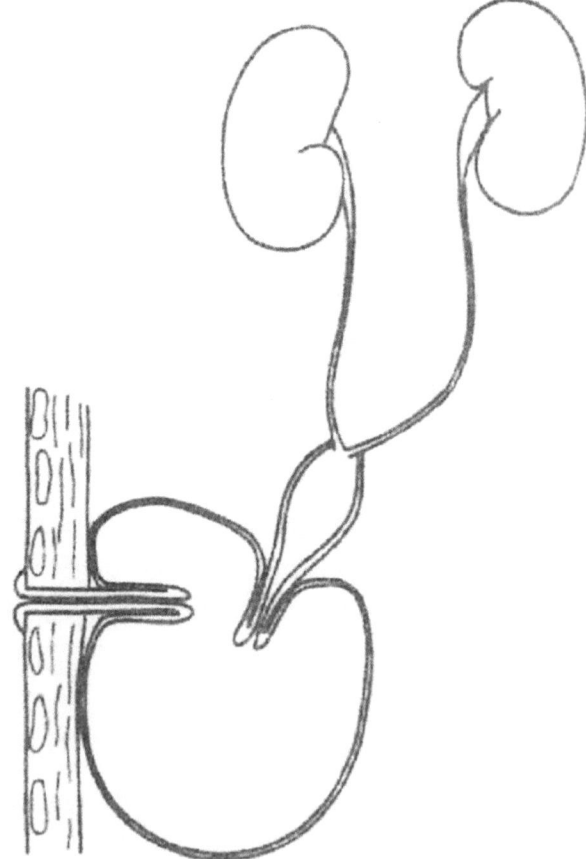

Fig. 1.15 Continent ileal reservoir for cutaneous urinary deviation. The ureters are connected to the reservoir via a reflux preventing nipple valve. (Åkerlund S, Berglund B, Granerus G, Jensen J, Kock NG, Philipson B. Drainage of the Upper Urinary Tract as recorded with Renography in Patients with a Continent Urostomy (Kock Pouch). Scand J Urol Nephrol. 1987;21:109–114. Copyright Acta Chirurgica Scandinavian Society, reprinted by permission of Taylor & Francis on behalf of Acta Chirurgica Scandinavia Society.)

gained popularity during the 1980s and 1990s together with other types of cutaneous urinary diversion [59]. Due to the complexity of the operation and the postoperative morbidity as well as the need for reoperations in 10–20% of the patients [60], the Kock pouch urinary reservoir has become less attractive, but is still an option for continent urostomy diversion [61–65].

During the late 1980s, Kock together with professor Ghoneim in Egypt developed methods to overcome the problems of cystectomy for Bilharzia and bladder cancer using the ileal pouch as orthotopic substitute for the bladder [66, 67]. Based on the earlier experiences with the orthotropic bladder substitute and the continent urostomy, they sutured the ileal pouch with a reflux-preventing valve to the ureter. In a way, this closes the circle from studies on bladder substitutes to continent ileostomy and finally continent urostomy and orthotropic bladder substitution.

1.5   Ileal Pouch Anal Anastomosis

The popularity of the continent ileostomy was in its heights in the 1970s and the early 1980s [68]. After introduction of the ileal pouch-anal anastomosis in 1980, this operation has become the method of choice for most patients with Ulcerative Colitis or Familial Polyposis who face proctocolectomy. The continent ileostomy has lost its importance in most places today [41, 69].

However, the long term results imply that the ileal pouch-anal anastomosis may not be the panacea it was initially thought to be [70]. The cumulative risk for pouch failure failure rate appears to be about 10% over 10 years [71–79]. Pelvic sepsis, poor function and pouchitis in that order seem to be the main reasons for failures.

According to reports in the literature, pouch excision with construction of a conventional ileostomy appears to the most common measure employed for these patients - a very unfortunate decision however as such an operation will unevitably be associated with loss of a significant length of terminal ileum. Apart from the practical problems of a high-flow ileostomy, salt-water imbalance and malabsorbtion of bile acids and vitamin B12 will develop.

Excision is particularly unfortunate as the failed ileal pouch-anal anastomosis may be converted to a continent ileostomy [80–87] - a technical demanding but often beneficial procedure worthwhile for motivated patients. It seems reasonable to assume that there may well be a great revival of interest in the continent ileostomy technique in the future.

1.6   Concluding Remarks

Since the early 1970s, thousands of patients have benefited from the invention of the continent ileostomy offering the patients an improved quality of life. The excellent health of the majority of the patients with continent ileostomy, some of them observed for more than 20 years, confirms the safety of the procedure. Kock reservoir for urinary diversion and orthotopic bladder substitution further indicate the importance of this ingenious invention.

The history of the continent ileostomy is a story about invention, studies in physiology and pathophysiology aimed at improvements of the method and application of meticulous surgical technique. It is the story of a remarkable scientific achievement starting with studies on urinary bladder substitutes and construction of a low pressure ileal reservoir for urinary bladder replacement, the development of the continent ileostomy reservoir for collection of faeces and finally the continent urostomy for urinary diversion. The concept of the Kock continent ileostomy radically changed the surgical concept of faecal diversion and pawed the way for the ileal pouch-anal anastomosis.

Bibliography

1. Bricker EM. Bladder substitution after pelvic evisceration. Surg Clin North Am. 1950;30(5):1511–21.
2. Bricker EM, Eiseman B. Bladder reconstruction from cecum and ascending colon following resection of pelvic viscera. Ann Surg. 1950;132(1):77–84.
3. Tasker JH. Ileo-cystoplasty: a new technique; an experimental study with report of a case. Br J Urol. 1953;25(4):349–57.
4. Giertz G, Franksson C. Construction of a substitute bladder, with preservation of urethral voiding, after subtotal and total cystectomy. Acta Chir Scand. 1957;113(3):218–28.
5. Kock NG. An experimental analysis of mechanisms engaged in reflex inhibition of intestinal motility. Acta Physiol Scand Suppl. 1959;47(164):1–54.
6. Faxen A, Kock NG, Sundin T. Long-term functional results after ileocystoplasty. Scand J Urol Nephrol. 1973;7(2):127–30.
7. Kock NG. Intra-abdominal "reservoir" in patients with permanent ileostomy. Preliminary observations on a procedure resulting in fecal "continence" in five ileostomy patients. Arch Surg. 1969;99(2):223–31.
8. Kock NG, Darle N, Hulten L, Kewenter J, Myrvold H, Philipson B. Ileostomy. Curr Probl Surg. 1977;14(8):1–52.
9. Kock NG. Continent ileostomy. Prog Surg. 1973;12:180–201.
10. Steichen FM. The creation of autologous substitute organs with stapling instruments. Am J Surg. 1977;134(5):659–73.
11. Kock NG, Brevinge H, Philipson BM, Ojerskog B. Continent ileostomy. The present technique and long term results. Ann Chir Gynaecol. 1986;75(2):63–70.
12. Gelernt IM, Bauer JJ, Kreel I. The reservoir ileostomy: early experience with 54 patients. Ann Surg. 1977;185(2):179–84.
13. Barnett WO. Modified techniques for improving the continent ileostomy. Am Surg. 1984;50(2):66–9.
14. Barnett WO. Current experiences with the continent intestinal reservoir. Surg Gynecol Obstet. 1989;168(1):1–5.
15. Kaiser AM, Stein JP, Beart RW Jr. T-pouch: a new valve design for a continent ileostomy. Dis Colon Rectum. 2002;45(3):411–5.
16. Kaiser AM. T-pouch: results of the first 10 years with a nonintussuscepting continent ileostomy. Dis Colon Rectum. 2012;55(2):155–62.
17. Berglund B, Kock NG, Myrvold HE. Volume capacity and pressure characteristics of the continent cecal reservoir. Surg Gynecol Obstet. 1986;163(1):42–8.

18. Berglund B, Kock NG. Volume capacity and pressure characteristics of various types of intestinal reservoirs. World J Surg. 1987;11(6):798–803.
19. Gadacz TR, Kelly KA, Phillips SF. The continent ileal pouch: absorptive and motor features. Gastroenterology. 1977;72(6):1287–91.
20. Hahnloser P, Sauberli H, Geroulanos S, Schauwecker HH, Kock NG. Continent ileostomyDOUBLEHYPHENindication and possibilities. Schweiz Med Wochenschr. 1975;105(25): 800–4.
21. Sauberli H, Geroulanos S, Hahnloser P, Schauwecker H, Kock NG. Studies of the dynamics of the "nipple valve" in dogs with continent colostomies. Dis Colon Rectum. 1974;17(6):735–40.
22. Myrvold HE, Jonsson KO. Pressure profiles in ileal pouch outlets. Scand J Gastroenterol. 1979;14(6):753–9.
23. Halvorsen JF, Heimann P, Hoel R, Nygaard K. The continent reservoir ileostomy: review of a collective series of thirty-six patients from three surgical departments. Surgery. 1978;83(3):252–8.
24. Schjonsby H, Halvorsen JF, Hofstad T, Hovdenak N. Stagnant loop syndrome in patients with continent ileostomy (intra-abdominal ileal reservoir). Gut. 1977;18(10):795–9.
25. Kelley DG, Branon ME, Phillips SF, Kelly KA. Diarrhoea after continent ileostomy. Gut. 1980;21(8):711–6.
26. Kay RM, Cohen Z, Siu KP, Petrunka CN, Strasberg SM. Ileal excretion and bacterial modification of bile acids and cholesterol in patients with continent ileostomy. Gut. 1980;21(2):128–32.
27. Brandberg A, Kock NG, Philipson B. Bacterial flora in intraabdominal ileostomy reservoir. A study of 23 patients provided with "continent ileostomy". Gastroenterology. 1972;63(3):413–6.
28. Philipson B, Brandberg A, Jagenburg R, Kock NG, Lager I, Ahren C. Mucosal morphology, bacteriology, and absorption in intra-abdominal ileostomy reservoir. Scand J Gastroenterol. 1975;10(2):145–53.
29. Nilsson LO, Andersson H, Hulten L, Jagenburg R, Kock NG, Myrvold HE, et al. Absorption studies in patients six to 10 years after construction of ileostomy reservoirs. Gut. 1979;20(6):499–503.
30. Ojerskog B, Kock NG, Nilsson LO, Philipson BM, Ahren C. Long-term follow-up of patients with continent ileostomies. Dis Colon Rectum. 1990;33(3):184–9.
31. Nilsson LO, Myrvold HE, Swolin B, Ojerskog B. Vitamin B12 in plasma in patients with continent ileostomy and long observation time. Scand J Gastroenterol. 1984;19(3):369–74.
32. Nilsson LO, Kock NG, Lindgren I, Myrvold HE, Philipson BM, Ahren C. Morphological and histochemical changes in the mucosa of the continent ileostomy reservoir 6DOUBLEHYPHEN10 years after its construction. Scand J Gastroenterol. 1980;15(6):737–47.
33. Nilsson LO, Andersson H, Bosaeus I, Myrvold HE. Total body water and total body potassium in patients with continent ileostomies. Gut. 1982;23(7):589–93.
34. Andersson H, Fasth S, Filipsson S, Hellberg R, Hulten L, Nilsson LO, et al. Faecal excretion of intravenously injected 14C-cholic acid in patients with conventional ileostomy and in patients with continent ileostomy reservoir. Scand J Gastroenterol. 1979;14(5):551–4.
35. Brevinge H, Berglund B, Kock NG. Ileostomy output of gas and feces before and after conversion from conventional to reservoir ileostomy. Dis Colon Rectum. 1992;35(7):662–9.
36. Kock NG, Myrvold HE, Nilsson LO. Progress report on the continent ileostomy. World J Surg. 1980;4(2):143–8.
37. Kock NG, Myrvold HE, Nilsson LO, Philipson BM. Continent ileostomy. An account of 314 patients. Acta Chir Scand. 1981;147(1):67–72.
38. Kock NG, Myrvold HE, Nilsson LO, Philipson BM. 18 years' experience with continent ileostomy. Chirurg. 1985;56(5):299–304.
39. Kock NG. Continent ileostomy. In: Allgöver Bseryc M, Gruber UF, editors. Progress in surgery, vol. 12. Basel: S.Karger, Basel; 1973. p. 180–201.
40. Myrvold HE, Kock NG. Continent ileostomy in inflammatory bowel disease. In: Jerzy Glass PS GB, editor. Progress in gastroenterology. IV. New York: Grune & Stratton; 1983. p. 311–23.
41. Hulten L. Proctocolectomy and ileostomy to pouch surgery for ulcerative colitis. World J Surg. 1998;22(4):335–41.

42. Kiran RP, Remzi FH, Fazio VW, Lavery IC, Church JM, Strong SA, et al. Complications and functional results after ileoanal pouch formation in obese patients. J Gastrointest Surg. 2008;12(4):668–74.

43. Ecker KW. The continent ileostomy. Current indications, techniques and results. Chirurg. 1999;70(6):635–42.

44. Fazio VW, Church JM. Complications and function of the continent ileostomy at the Cleveland Clinic. World J Surg. 1988;12(2):148–54.

45. Jarvinen HJ, Makitie A, Sivula A. Long-term results of continent ileostomy. Int J Color Dis. 1986;1(1):40–3.

46. Lepisto AH, Jarvinen HJ. Durability of Kock continent ileostomy. Dis Colon Rectum. 2003;46(7):925–8.

47. Nessar G, Wu JS. Evolution of continent ileostomy. World J Gastroenterol. 2012;18(27):3479–82.

48. Litle VR, Barbour S, Schrock TR, Welton ML. The continent ileostomy: long-term durability and patient satisfaction. J Gastrointest Surg. 1999;3(6):625–32.

49. Wasmuth HH, Svinsas M, Trano G, Rydning A, Endreseth BH, Wibe A, et al. Surgical load and long-term outcome for patients with Kock continent ileostomy. Color Dis. 2007;9(8):713–7.

50. Dozois RR, Kelly KA, Beart RW Jr, Beahrs OH. Improved results with continent ileostomy. Ann Surg. 1980;192(3):319–24.

51. Svaninger G, Nordgren S, Oresland T, Hulten L. Incidence and characteristics of pouchitis in the Kock continent ileostomy and the pelvic pouch. Scand J Gastroenterol. 1993;28(8):695–700.

52. Parks AG, Nicholls RJ. Proctocolectomy without ileostomy for ulcerative colitis. Br Med J. 1978;2(6130):85–8.

53. Parks AG, Nicholls RJ, Belliveau P. Proctocolectomy with ileal reservoir and anal anastomosis. Br J Surg. 1980;67(8):533–8.

54. Kock NG, Hulten L, Myrvold HE. Ileoanal anastomosis with interposition of the ileal 'Kock pouch'. Preliminary results. Dis Colon Rectum. 1989;32(12):1050–4.

55. Trasti H. Urinary diversion via a continent ileum reservoir. An experimental and clinical study. Scand J Urol Nephrol Suppl. 1978;(49):1–71.

56. Kock NG, Nilson AE, Nilsson LO, Norlen LJ, Philipson BM. Urinary diversion via a continent ileal reservoir: clinical results in 12 patients. J Urol. 1982;128(3):469–75.

57. Jonsson O, Olofsson G, Lindholm E, Tornqvist H. Long-time experience with the Kock ileal reservoir for continent urinary diversion. Eur Urol. 2001;40(6):632–40.

58. Berglund B, Brevinge H, Akerlund S, Kock NG. Significance of the antireflux valve for upper urinary tract pressure. An experimental study in patients with urinary diversion via a continent ileal reservoir. Scand J Urol Nephrol. 1992;26(1):29–33.

59. Skinner DG, Lieskovsky G, Boyd SD. Continuing experience with the continent ileal reservoir (Kock pouch) as an alternative to cutaneous urinary diversion: an update after 250 cases. J Urol. 1987;137(6):1140–5.

60. Skinner DG, Boyd SD, Lieskovsky G. An update on the Kock pouch for continent urinary diversion. Urol Clin North Am. 1987;14(4):789–95.

61. Skinner EC. Continent cutaneous diversion. Curr Opin Urol. 2015;25(6):555–61.

62. Nieh PT. The Kock pouch urinary reservoir. Urol Clin North Am. 1997;24(4):755–72.

63. Hautmann R. Urinary diversion 1989. Urologe A. 1989;28(4):177–82.

64. Lee RK, Abol-Enein H, Artibani W, Bochner B, Dalbagni G, Daneshmand S, et al. Urinary diversion after radical cystectomy for bladder cancer: options, patient selection, and outcomes. BJU Int. 2014;113(1):11–23.

65. Pycha A, Burger M, Palermo S. Urinary diversion: tailored solutions for individual patients. Curr Opin Urol. 2015;25(5):436–40.

66. Ghoneim MA, Kock NG, Lycke G, El-Din AB. An appliance-free, sphincter-controlled bladder substitute: the urethral Kock pouch. J Urol. 1987;138(5):1150–4.

67. Kock NG, Ghoneim MA, Lycke KG, Mahran MR. Replacement of the bladder by the urethral Kock pouch: functional results, urodynamics and radiological features. J Urol. 1989;141(5):1111–6.

68. Hulten L, Svaninger G. Facts about the Kock continent ileostomy. Dis Colon Rectum. 1984;27(8):553–7.
69. Hulten L. The continent ileostomy (Kock's pouch) versus the restorative proctocolectomy (pelvic pouch). World J Surg. 1985;9(6):952–9.
70. Hulten L, Fasth S, Hallgren T, Oresland T. The failing pelvic pouch conversion to continent ileostomy. Int J Color Dis. 1992;7(3):119–21.
71. Fazio VW, Ziv Y, Church JM, Oakley JR, Lavery IC, Milsom JW, et al. Ileal pouch-anal anastomoses complications and function in 1005 patients. Ann Surg. 1995;222(2):120–7.
72. Tulchinsky H, Hawley PR, Nicholls J. Long-term failure after restorative proctocolectomy for ulcerative colitis. Ann Surg. 2003;238(2):229–34.
73. Hahnloser D, Pemberton JH, Wolff BG, Larson DR, Crownhart BS, Dozois RR. Results at up to 20 years after ileal pouch-anal anastomosis for chronic ulcerative colitis. Br J Surg. 2007;94(3):333–40.
74. Tekkis PP, Lovegrove RE, Tilney HS, Smith JJ, Sagar PM, Shorthouse AJ, et al. Long-term failure and function after restorative proctocolectomy - a multi-centre study of patients from the UK National Ileal Pouch Registry. Color Dis. 2010;12(5):433–41.
75. Wasmuth HH, Trano G, Endreseth B, Rydning A, Wibe A, Myrvold HE. Long-term surgical load in patients with ileal pouch-anal anastomosis. Color Dis. 2009;11(7):711–8.
76. Rokke O, Iversen K, Olsen T, Ristesund SM, Eide GE, Turowski GE. Long-term followup with evaluation of the surgical and functional results of the ileal pouch reservoir in restorative proctocolectomy for ulcerative colitis. ISRN Gastroenterol. 2011;2011:625842.
77. Mark-Christensen A, Erichsen R, Brandsborg S, Ronne Pachler F, Norager CB, Johansen N, et al. Pouch failures following ileal pouch-anal anastomosis for ulcerative colitis. Colorectal Dis. 2017.
78. Belliveau P, Trudel J, Vasilevsky CA, Stein B, Gordon PH. Ileoanal anastomosis with reservoirs: complications and long-term results. Can J Surg. 1999;42(5):345–52.
79. Yu CS, Pemberton JH, Larson D. Ileal pouch-anal anastomosis in patients with indeterminate colitis: long-term results. Dis Colon Rectum. 2000;43(11):1487–96.
80. Borjesson L, Oresland T, Hulten L. The failed pelvic pouch: conversion to a continent ileostomy. Tech Coloproctol. 2004;8(2):102–5.
81. Wasmuth HH, Trano G, Wibe A, Endreseth BH, Rydning A, Myrvold HE. Failed pelvic pouch substituted by continent ileostomy. Color Dis. 2010;12(7 Online):e109–13.
82. Lian LF, Dietz V, Remzi D, Shen F, Wu B, Kiran R. Outcomes after conversion of failed Ileal Pouch-Anal Anastomosis (IPAA) to Continent Ileostomy (CI) in a Single Tertiary Center. Dis Colon Rectum. 2008;51(5):2.
83. Wassmuth HH, Myrvold HE, Bengtsson J, Hulten L. Conversion of a failed pouch to a continent ileostomy: a controversy. Color Dis. 2011;13(1):2–5.
84. Kusunoki M, Sakanoue Y, Shoji Y, Kusuhara K, Yamamura T, Utsunomiya J. Conversion of malfunctioning J pouch to Kock's pouch. Case report. Acta Chir Scand. 1990;156(2):179–81.
85. Ecker KW, Haberer M, Feifel G. Conversion of the failing ileoanal pouch to reservoir-ileostomy rather than to ileostomy alone. Dis Colon Rectum. 1996;39(9):977–80.
86. Castillo E, Thomassie LM, Whitlow CB, Margolin DA, Malcolm J, Beck DE. Continent ileostomy: current experience. Dis Colon Rectum. 2005;48(6):1263–8.
87. Behrens DT, Paris M, Luttrell JN. Conversion of failed ileal pouch-anal anastomosis to continent ileostomy. Dis Colon Rectum. 1999;42(4):490–5. discussion 5–6.

Chapter 2
Indications

Thomas Hallgren

2.1 Ulcerative Colitis

Until the early 1970s proctocolectomy and a terminal ileostomy was the gold standard for operative treatment of ulcerative colitis.

During the 1960s professor Nils Kock in Gothenburg developed the continent ileostomy, utilising the terminal ileum for the construction of a continent intraabdominal reservoir after proctocolectomy for Ulcerative Colitis. The continent ileostomy or the Kock pouch was introduced as the first alternative for patients wishing to avoid a permanent ileostomy after this procedure [1]. Several modifications of the technique were made in the following years. After adding a nipple construction to achieve continence, the main features of the Kock pouch were in place as still in use today. An initial publication on the results of the continent ileostomy was made from Kock in 1973 [2]. Thereafter the technique was spread and adopted by a number of colorectal surgeons around the world. The operation eliminated the need for external appliances and improved the quality of life for many patients [3–5]. However, it's spread was limited due to the complexity of the procedure and the relatively frequent need for revisional surgery. A more extensive presentation of the development and the technical details of pouch construction are given in Chaps. 1 and 5.

In 1978 Parks and Nicholls were the first to publish a series of patients operated with total proctocolectomy, endoanal mucosectomy and reconstruction with an ileal reservoir anastomosed to the remaining anal canal – the ileal pouch-anal anastomosis [6]. This technique revolutionised the operative treatment of Inflammatory Bowel Disease and familial adenomatous polyposis by omitting the need of a permanent stoma and preserving the normal route of defecation. In the subsequent years, it was gradually adopted by most highly specialised colorectal units around the world, and

T. Hallgren (✉)
Department of Surgery, Central Hospital, Karlstad, Sweden

© Springer Nature Switzerland AG 2019
P. Myrelid, M. Block (eds.), *The Kock Pouch*,
https://doi.org/10.1007/978-3-319-95591-9_2

is today considered as the method of choice in restorative proctocolectomy for Ulcerative Colitis and Familial Adenomatous Polyposis. Several studies have shown a normal quality of life in patients operated with a pelvic pouch [7, 8].

As more and more referral centres within inflammatory bowel disease gained experience with the pelvic pouch, the use of the Kock pouch declined. Today only a limited number of surgeons with a large experience of the technique can be found in practice. There is, however, still a place for the continent ileostomy in the surgical armamentarium. The indications today are relatively few, but surgeons and gastro-enterologists, caring for patients with inflammatory bowel disease and Familial Adenomatous Polyposis must have a basic knowledge about the procedure, it's indications and complications to be able to counsel their patients correctly and wisely when surgery is needed. As the procedure is complex, it is today centralized to highly specialized colorectal centres - in Sweden two institutions.

Pelvic pouch construction should always be performed as a planned procedure, either together with proctocolectomy, or after a previous colectomy and in conjunction to a proctectomy. Two important prerequisites for a successful pelvic pouch construction are needed; a well-functioning anal sphincter and a sufficient small bowel length to make it possible to join the apex of the pouch with the anal canal without tension.

Pouch function is closely related to anal sphincter function and it is therefore vital to assess the sphincter function before pelvic pouch construction, especially since the operation itself tends to impair the sphincter [9, 10]. Anal sphincter function may be divided into two separate entities: the resting anal pressure and the maximal squeeze pressure. Resting anal pressure is mainly maintained by the action of the internal anal sphincter – a smooth muscle, whereas maximal squeeze pressure is generated by contraction of the striated external anal sphincter. Trauma with following sphincter dysfunction can affect either one or both of these muscles. Obstetric trauma is the most common cause, but anal surgical procedures and accidents to the perineal area can negatively affect sphincter function. Neurological disease is another reason for sphincter dysfunction that should not be forgotten or overlooked.

A careful history regarding any degree of faecal incontinence, and in women also previous obstetric complications, must be taken before a pelvic pouch operation. A thorough digital anal examination should always be undertaken. If sphincter dysfunction is in any way suspected, further evaluations, such as anal manometry and ultrasound examination should be performed. If sphincter dysfunction is shown, expected functional outcome must be evaluated and discussed with the patient together with other surgical alternatives, of which the construction of a Kock pouch is one possibility.

Small bowel reach cannot normally be judged preoperatively, but is in rare cases experienced during surgery when intending to construct a pelvic pouch. Severe adhesions or just a short mesentery can be possible causes. If surgical procedures, such as incision of the mesentery, cannot solve the problem the construction of a Kock pouch may be a possible solution, either directly or later, depending on the information given to the patient beforehand.

Thus, a few clinical scenarios remain where a Koch pouch may be an alternative for patients with Ulcerative Colitis.

Indications today for Kock pouch construction in patients with Ulcerative Colitis

- As primary procedure;

  - In patients with impairment of anal sphincter function making a pelvic pouch not feasible.
  - In patients with insufficient small bowel reach making the ileal-anal anastomosis impossible during intended pelvic pouch construction.

- As secondary procedure;

  - After pelvic pouch failure – further discussed in Chap. 6.

2.2 Indeterminate Colitis

Indeterminate colitis is defined as histopathologic findings after colectomy for inflammatory bowel disease with overlapping and mixed features of Ulcerative Colitis and Crohn's disease, making a certain distinction between the two entities impossible. It is found in an average of 5% of inflammatory bowel disease colectomies, but varies between reports from 1–20% [11]. Over time the majority of patients remain with a diagnosis of indeterminate colitis, or show symptoms similar to Ulcerative Colitis [12]. Only a small portion will develop signs or manifestations of Crohn's disease.

In a large study from Nessar et al. five out of 330 patients (1.5%) operated with a Kock pouch had indeterminate colitis as preoperative diagnosis [4]. The small number of patients with indeterminate colitis in this and other studies presenting outcome after the construction of a Kock pouch does not allow any meaningful comparison between this group of patients and those with other diagnoses.

Studies on patients with indeterminate colitis operated with an ileal pouch-anal anastomosis have shown that there were more pouch-related complications (mainly fistula formation) in patients with indeterminate colitis compared to those with Ulcerative Colitis. However, function and survival of the pouch, as well as quality of life, were similar in the two groups [13, 14].

The natural history of indeterminate colitis more closely resembles Ulcerative Colitis than that of Crohn's disease, and it has not so far been possible to beforehand distinguish patients with a higher risk for Crohn's disease development over time.

With this in mind, together with the above findings from pelvic pouch surgery, it is reasonable to inform and treat patients with indeterminate colitis, and without any clinical manifestation of Crohn's disease, according to the same principles as for Ulcerative Colitis when considering the construction of a Kock pouch.

The indications for construction of a Kock pouch in patients with indeterminate colitis, therefore, are the same as above stated for Ulcerative Colitis.

2.3   Crohn's Disease

Crohn's disease may involve any part of the gastrointestinal tract, including a pouch constructed of the terminal ileum. Many surgeons as well as gastroenterologists, therefore, consider Crohn's disease as being a contraindication to pouch construction. Even so, pouch procedures, Kock pouch as well as pelvic pouch, have been performed in patients with Crohn's disease. In the early reports Kock pouch was used as a primary procedure after proctocolectomy for Crohn's disease. The results were disappointing with recurrent disease in a substantial number of pouches within the first year after surgery [15–17]. Based on these experiences the authors recommended that the Kock pouch should not be performed in patients with Crohn's disease. However, these patients were not subjected to any specific selection procedures and often retrospectively diagnosed with active small bowel disease.

According to these reports the strategies for Crohn's disease and pouch surgery changed in many units. The hypothesis was that well selected patients would result in a better outcome. Patients considered for a Kock pouch were those with Crohn's disease confined to the colon and rectum (without any small bowel engagement) or patients with a longer disease-free interval of 5–10 years after proctocolectomy and a Brooke ileostomy.

Crohn's disease of the pouch may however later develop, months to years after pouch construction, even though small bowel Crohn's disease had been ruled out preoperatively. This may be true even if the proctocolectomy specimen after surgery did not show any evident clinical or histopathological signs of Crohn's disease. An alternative explanation is that operative changes of bowel anatomy may trigger development of Crohn's disease. Such an explanation is supported by clinical findings that most Crohn lesions in pouch patients are located at the anastomosis or at bowel segments just proximal to it [18].

In a recent report from the Cleveland Clinic 48 patients with a final diagnosis of Crohn's disease were identified among all patients operated with a Kock pouch between 1978 and 2013 [19]. The diagnosis of Crohn's disease was made before construction of the Kock pouch in 15 patients and in 33 patients at a later stage. Major revisions were performed in 40 patients and minor in 13 patients. Valve-related problems, such as slippage and prolapse, as well as pouchitis were the most frequently encountered complications. During long-term follow-up failure of the Kock pouch was similar irrespective of if the diagnosis of Crohn's disease was made pre- or post-operatively. Kaplan-Meier estimates showed a Kock pouch survival of 79% at five and 48% at 20 years. Five patients developed short-bowel syndrome.

Even if medical treatment can improve pouch survival the results must be considered as relatively poor. Still it is important to point out that patients with a Kock pouch in function, even after one or several revisions, are generally very satisfied with their quality of life and prepared to endure even further procedures to save their pouch. A post-operative diagnosis of Crohn's disease as such does not mandate an excision of the Kock pouch.

Reports from series of patients with Crohn's disease and operated with a pelvic pouch have shown an overall long-term pouch retention rate of 71% at 10 years [20]. Results were significantly worse for patients with a delayed diagnosis of Crohn's disease compared to those diagnosed before or at surgery. At the end of the day, this implies that a substantial number of patients with a pelvic pouch and a final diagnosis of Crohn's disease will require additional surgery where a Kock pouch is one possible alternative.

Based on these findings and clinical experiences many pouch surgeons today consider that a few indications remain as acceptably safe alternatives for constructing a Kock pouch in well selected patients with Crohn's disease.

Indications today for Kock pouch construction in patients with Crohn's disease

- As primary procedure;

  - Together with proctocolectomy for Crohn's disease confined to the colon and rectum, in patients not feasible for pelvic pouch (usually due to perianal disease).

- As secondary procedure;

  - After previous proctocolectomy in patients with a terminal ileostomy severely affecting their quality of life, and with a disease-free interval of at least 5 years.
  - In patients operated with a pelvic pouch developing pouch complications (mainly fistula formation) due to a final diagnosis of Crohn's disease requiring re-operation and where a redo-procedure is not an alternative.

It must be pointed out that preoperative investigations to rule out small bowel Crohn's disease in all circumstances must be extensive, including clinical and laboratory investigations, endoscopy and radiology, favourably magnetic resonance imaging or capsule endoscopy.

The most feared risk over lifetime in Crohn's disease patients is disease recurrence, requiring repeated bowel resections with the risk of developing short-bowel syndrome. A thorough follow-up and early identification and treatment of disease recurrence in this group of patients is therefore of utmost importance. This should be undertaken by a team of experienced surgeons and gastroenterologists working in close co-operation.

2.4 Familial Adenomatous Polyposis

Familial Adenomatous Polyposis is a hereditary disease with the formation of multiple adenomatous polyps in the colon and rectum [21, 22]. The classic type of Familial Adenomatous Polyposis is an autosomal dominantly inherited disease that accounts for approximately 1% of all colorectal cancer cases and has a prevalence of approximately 1 in 10,000. The number of polyps increases with age, and hundreds to thousands of polyps can develop in the colon and rectum. A milder type of Familial Adenomatous Polyposis, called autosomal recessive Familial Adenomatous Polyposis, has also been identified. People with the autosomal recessive type of this disorder develop fewer polyps than those with the classic type.

Polyps may start to develop as early as in the adolescent years. Even though the polyps are initially non-malignant, they will almost invariably become malignant over time. Patients with the classic type of Familial Adenomatous Polyposis have an almost 100% risk of developing colorectal cancer. The average age of onset of polyposis in Familial Adenomatous Polyposis is 16 years, whereas the average age of onset for colorectal cancer in this group is 39 years. Prophylactic surgery before progression to malignancy is recommended as the treatment of choice. In virtually all cases a proctocolectomy is needed. An often recommended age for this operative procedure is 20 years of age [23].

High-grade dysplasia in mucosal biopsies may require earlier intervention and of course also the development of a manifest colorectal carcinoma. In the latter case the treatment strategies are different and according to oncological principles.

Since the introduction of the pelvic pouch in the early 1980s this procedure has become the gold standard for restorative proctocolectomy in patients with Familial Adenomatous Polyposis. The remaining indication for a Kock pouch has been those not suitable for a pelvic pouch.

No series of patients operated for Familial Adenomatous Polyposis with a proctocolectomy and a continent ileostomy and thereafter separately followed can be found in the literature. In most series, their outcome has been evaluated together with patients operated for Ulcerative Colitis. In the large series of Kock pouch construction from Nessar et al. [4], comprising 330 patients, 23 patients (7%) were operated for Familial Adenomatous Polyposis and 251 patients for Ulcerative Colitis. The whole group had a functioning pouch in 87% after 10 years and 77% after 20 years. However, two Familial Adenomatous Polyposis patients died of rectal cancer!

Another problem for patients with Familial Adenomatous Polyposis is the risk for development of desmoid tumours. Desmoids are rare, benign fibromatous lesions that most frequently arise in the abdominal wall and/or mesentery but can also occasionally develop in the extremities and trunk. A study from Johns Hopkins University showed that 10% of Familial Adenomatous Polyposis patients developed a desmoid [24].

Depending on the site of growth and their size, they may limit small bowel reach, or narrow the small pelvis, making pelvic pouch construction impossible. In such cases a Kock pouch may be an alternative.

Indications today for Kock pouch construction in patients with Familial Adenomatous Polyposis

- As primary procedure;
  - Together with proctocolectomy for Familial Adenomatous Polyposis when pelvic pouch is not feasible due to either;
    - anal sphincter dysfunction
    - insufficient small bowel reach

- early carcinoma involving the anorectum and therefore requiring a complete resection of the region, or
- desmoid development in the abdominal cavity or small pelvis making IPAA impossible.

- As secondary procedure;

  - In patients with pelvic pouch for Familial Adenomatous Polyposis with pouch complications requiring re-operation and where a re-do procedure is not an alternative.

Follow-up strategies and surveillance after Kock pouch is discussed in Chap. 12. Regarding patients with Familial Adenomatous Polyposis follow-up must be remembered in the long-term, in particular due the well-known risk for malignant polyp formation and cancer development in the upper gastrointestinal tract [25]. The risk for desmoid formation seems to increase after surgical procedures and give cause for regular follow-up.

2.5 The Failed Pelvic Pouch

Failure of a pelvic pouch may be defined as the need for pouch excision, or having a permanent pouch diversion with a proximal loop-ileostomy. Depending on the reason of pouch failure the conversion of a pelvic pouch into a continent ileostomy may be possible and was early described by Hultén et al. [26]. The technique for conversion is described in Chap. 6.

Due to the large overall number of patients operated with a pelvic pouch, and with a reported failure rate of 10–15%, it is possible that in the future pelvic pouch failure may become the single most frequent indication for construction of a continent ileostomy [27, 28].

2.6 Other Diagnoses

Other diagnoses, such as colonic inertia, Hirschsprung's disease, rectal villous adenoma and imperforate anus, have been reported being operated with a Kock pouch [4]. There is, however, no follow-up available for these rare indications and the outcome therefore not possible to further comment on.

We believe that Kock pouch may still be a possible alternative in seldom occurring cases where a terminal ileostomy is the only remaining option and when the patient has a strong wish to avoid it. Individual information and counselling in a co-operation with an experienced stoma nurse is then of absolute importance.

References

1. Kock N. Intra-abdominal "reservoir" in patients with permanent ileostomy. Arch Surg. 1969;99:223–31.
2. Kock NG. Continent ileostomy. Prog Surg. 1973;12:180–201.
3. Ojerskog B, Hallstrom T, Kock NG, Myrvold HE. Quality of life in ileostomy patients before and after conversion to the continent ileostomy. Int J Color Dis. 1988;3(3):166–70.
4. Nessar G, Fazio VW, Tekkis P, Connor J, Wu J, Bast J, et al. Long-term outcome and quality of life after continent ileostomy. Dis Colon Rectum. 2006;49(3):336–44.
5. Berndtsson IE, Lindholm E, Oresland T, Hulten L. Health-related quality of life and pouch function in continent ileostomy patients: a 30-year perspective. Dis Colon Rectum. 2004;47(12):2131–7.
6. Parks AG, Nicholls RJ. Proctocolectomy without ileostomy for ulcerative colitis. Br Med J. 1978;2(6130):85–8.
7. Richards DM, Hughes SA, Irving MH, Scott NA. Patient quality of life after successful restorative proctocolectomy is normal. Color Dis. 2001;3(4):223–6.
8. Berndtsson I, Oresland T. Quality of life before and after proctocolectomy and IPAA in patients with ulcerative proctocolitis--a prospective study. Color Dis. 2003;5(2):173–9.
9. Scott NA, Pemberton JH, Barkel DC, Wolff BG. Anal and ileal pouch manometric measurements before ileostomy closure are related to functional outcome after ileal pouch-anal anastomosis. Br J Surg. 1989;76(6):613–6.
10. Cullen JJ, Kelly KA. Prospectively evaluating anal sphincter function after ileal pouch-anal canal anastomosis. Am J Surg. 1994;167(6):558–61.
11. Odze RD. A contemporary and critical appraisal of 'indeterminate colitis'. Mod Pathol. 2015;28(Suppl 1):S30–46.
12. Mitchell PJ, Rabau MY, Haboubi NY. Indeterminate colitis. Tech Coloproctol. 2007;11(2):91–6.
13. Jackson KL, Stocchi L, Duraes L, Rencuzogullari A, Bennett AE, Remzi FH. Long-term outcomes in indeterminate colitis patients undergoing ileal pouch-anal anastomosis: function, quality of life, and complications. J Gastrointest Surg. 2017;21(1):56–61.
14. Brown CJ, Maclean AR, Cohen Z, Macrae HM, O'Connor BI, McLeod RS. Crohn's disease and indeterminate colitis and the ileal pouch-anal anastomosis: outcomes and patterns of failure. Dis Colon Rectum. 2005;48(8):1542–9.
15. Beart RW Jr, Beahrs OH, Kelly KA, Dozois RR, Wolf SA. The continent ileostomy: a viable alternative. Mayo Clin Proc. 1979;54(10):643–5.
16. Kock NG, Myrvold HE, Nilsson LO, Philipson BM. Continent ileostomy. an account of 314 patients. Acta Chir Scand. 1981;147(1):67–72.
17. Handelsman JC, Gottlieb LM, Hamilton SR. Crohn's disease as a contraindication to Kock pouch (continent ileostomy). Dis Colon Rectum. 1993;36(9):840–3.
18. Whelan G, Farmer RG, Fazio VW, Goormastic M. Recurrence after surgery in Crohn's disease. Relationship to location of disease (clinical pattern) and surgical indication. Gastroenterology. 1985;88(6):1826–33.
19. Aytac E, Dietz DW, Ashburn J, Remzi FH. Long-term outcomes after continent ileostomy creation in patients with Crohn's disease. Dis Colon Rectum. 2017;60(5):508–13.
20. Melton GB, Fazio VW, Kiran RP, He J, Lavery IC, Shen B, et al. Long-term outcomes with ileal pouch-anal anastomosis and Crohn's disease: pouch retention and implications of delayed diagnosis. Ann Surg. 2008;248(4):608–16.
21. Scott RJ, Meldrum C, Crooks R, Spigelman AD, Kirk J, Tucker K, et al. Familial adenomatous polyposis: more evidence for disease diversity and genetic heterogeneity. Gut. 2001;48(4):508–14.
22. Gardner EJ. A genetic and clinical study of intestinal polyposis, a predisposing factor for carcinoma of the colon and rectum. Am J Hum Genet. 1951;3(2):167–76.
23. Mills SJ, Chapman PD, Burn J, Gunn A. Endoscopic screening and surgery for familial adenomatous polyposis: dangerous delays. Br J Surg. 1997;84(1):74–7.

24. Gurbuz AK, Giardiello FM, Petersen GM, Krush AJ, Offerhaus GJ, Booker SV, et al. Desmoid tumours in familial adenomatous polyposis. Gut. 1994;35(3):377–81.
25. Groves CJ, Saunders BP, Spigelman AD, Phillips RK. Duodenal cancer in patients with familial adenomatous polyposis (FAP): results of a 10 year prospective study. Gut. 2002;50(5):636–41.
26. Hulten L, Fasth S, Hallgren T, Oresland T. The failing pelvic pouch conversion to continent ileostomy. Int J Color Dis. 1992;7(3):119–21.
27. Ide S, Araki T, Okita Y, Kawamura M, Toiyama Y, Kobayashi M, et al. Outcome and functional prognosis of pelvic sepsis after ileal pouch-anal anastomosis in patients with ulcerative colitis. Surg Today. 2017;47(3):301–6.
28. Lorenzo G, Maurizio C, Maria LP, Tanzanu M, Silvio L, Mariangela P, et al. Ileal pouch-anal anastomosis 20 years later: is it still a good surgical option for patients with ulcerative colitis? Int J Color Dis. 2016;31(12):1835–43.

Chapter 3
Contraindications

Mattias Block

3.1 Crohn's disease

Crohn's disease is often described as a contraindication to the construction of a Kock pouch, but a consensus opinion is less definite. Some authors suggest that Crohn's disease should continue to be regarded as a firm contraindication to the Kock pouch. Since Crohn's disease affects the entire gastrointestinal tract, the risk for reactivation or recurrence of the disease is high in patients after surgery. The risk for complications after Kock pouch surgery is increased in patients with Crohn's disease and also the risk for failure of the pouch is much higher. Active regional enteritis is to be considered an absolute contraindication to the construction of a continent ileostomy.

Therefore, Crohn's disease should be actively sought out and excluded preoperatively, and it should be treated aggressively if it is discovered after surgery. If such a patient requires further surgery, the Kock pouch should be removed, according to many authors.

However, the benefits afforded a patient with a Kock pouch are substantial and warrant consideration in a selected group of patients with Crohn's disease whom are disease-free for a minimum of 5 years (or 10 years according to some authors). In this group of highly selected, well-informed patients, a Kock pouch can be considered but the increased risk of complications and failure must be taken into consideration and thoroughly discussed with the patient.

M. Block (✉)
Department of Surgery, Sahlgrenska University Hospital, University of Gothenburg,
Gothenburg, Sweden
e-mail: mattias.block@vgregion.se

© Springer Nature Switzerland AG 2019
P. Myrelid, M. Block (eds.), *The Kock Pouch*,
https://doi.org/10.1007/978-3-319-95591-9_3

3.2 Marginal Small Bowel Length

Patients that previously have had small bowel resections are at risk of ending up with short bowel syndrome and as a result, malnutrition.

Construction of the Kock pouch itself demands a small bowel length of 45 cm. If the Kock pouch or pelvic pouch fails and has to be removed, the patient could be at risk of short bowel syndrome. This is even more stressed if the continent reservoir is revised and ending up with construction of a new reservoir, demanding an additional length of 45 cm of small bowel.

3.3 Obesity

Obesity, especially morbid obesity, is a contraindication due to various reasons, mainly because of the fact that a voluminous abdominal wall is difficult to handle when constructing the outlet. There is a higher risk of valve slipping resulting in incontinence of the pouch. Also, a bulky mesentery can be very demanding in constructing both the pouch itself and most of all, the nipple. Patients should be firmly motivated to reduce weight and contact with dietitian should be strongly encouraged. Some centers are more demanding towards patients and do not accept patients for surgery if body mass index exceeds 30. However, a firm and definite agreement does not exist within the surgical society involved in pouch surgery.

3.4 Malnutrition

In general, malnutrition is considered to be a contraindication in elective colorectal surgery. This is especially true in benign diseases, and even more so for advanced reconstructive procedures such as a Kock pouch. It is essential that patients are well nourished and are fully capable of healing as well as recovering after such a complex procedure as a Kock pouch.

3.5 Abdominal Wall Problems

Obese patients with extensive abdominal walls are difficult to handle and should be regarded as contraindication to Kock pouch surgery (see Obesity above). Other problems with the abdominal wall such as hernias, skin infections, and multiple scarring after previous surgery, to name a few, should all be taken into consideration as this might affect the outcome after Kock pouch surgery. This is even more important if there is an abdominal wall problem in the lower quadrants where the outlet is placed (preferably on patients right side even if the left side can be used in selected cases).

3.6 Smoking

Smoking is a strong risk factor for complications in all kinds of surgery and even so in Kock pouch surgery. Cessation of smoking should therefore be suggested and stressed to all patients going through the procedure of a Kock pouch. Smoking should be considered as an absolute contraindication for Kock pouch surgery.

3.7 Medication

Corticosteroids increase surgical complications, especially doses >20 mg during >6 weeks. Preferably, patients should be completely free of corticosteroids before going through a Kock pouch procedure. Concerning treatment with immuno-modulators and/or biologicals, results from different studies yield conflicting results. Some studies found more septic complications in patients on treatment with infliximab while other studies failed to confirm this finding. As long as results from different studies remain conflicting, the standing recommendation is not to perform a single stage restorative procto-colectomy in patients with on-going biological treatment. Preoperative immune-modulating therapy do not increase the risk of postoperative complications and should therefore not be considered as a contraindi-cation for Kock pouch surgery.

3.8 Mental Incapability

It is important that patients understand the complexity of Kock pouch surgery.

The patients should be well informed as well as mentally prepared for the risk of undergoing revisional surgery. It is of outmost importance that the surgeon get consent from a very well-informed patient before the procedure is taking place. Patients must also have the ability to handle intubations. Incapability of understanding or grasping such important and vital information should be considered as a contraindi-cation to Kock pouch surgery. If there is the slightest doubt about this it is always good to postpone the decision and to have a multidisciplinary discussion regarding the situation.

3.9 Acute/Emergency Surgery

Patients undergoing acute surgery are not fit for reconstructive surgery of any kind in an acute setting due to their state of health, often including malnutrition, septicae-mia, high dose of corticosteroids etc. Therefore, Kock pouch surgery is naturally contraindicated in the acute setting.

3.10   Familiar Adenomatous Polyposis

In patients with Familiar Adenomatous Polyposis development of desmoids (a benign tumorous lesion of connective tissue) can develop in the mesentery, but most of all in the abdominal wall, making the creation of a Kock pouch more or less impossible. Therefore, desmoids, but not Familiar Adenomatous Polyposis, are a relative contraindication for Kock pouch surgery.

3.11   Age

Age limits are not established or considered as an absolute contraindication. However, most surgeons and authors more or less agree upon not to offer Kock pouch surgery to patients older than 60 years, mainly due to the expected long-term revision rate of 40–50%. Again, the final decision whether or not to perform Kock pouch surgery is up to the surgeon and the patient at hand.

3.12   Comorbidity

In patients with severe comorbidity such as congestive heart disease, chronic obstructive pulmonary disease, renal failure, dementia, and neuro-psychiatric disorders to mention some are all contra-indications for advanced reconstructive procedures for benign disease, such as Kock pouch surgery.

3.13   Portal Hypertension

This is a condition resulting from liver cirrhosis (mainly due to primary sclerosing cholangitis strongly related to Ulcerative Colitis) and as an effect patients form stoma varicose that can cause serious bleedings. Therefore, creating a Kock pouch is only considered appropriate if the only alternative is an end ileostomy.

3.14   Malignancy

Patients undergoing proctocolectomy due to malignant disease and ending up with an end ileostomy could be candidates for a Kock pouch later on. However, there are demands that the patient should be disease-free without any signs of local recurrence or systemic metastatic disease 3 years from primary surgery (in some centres and in some surgeons' opinions 5 years). So if the patient is disease-free after that follow-up time, creation of a Kock pouch could be taken into consideration.

Bibliography

1. Handelsman JC, Gottlieb LM, Hamilton SR. A reappraisal of the Kock continent ileostomy in patients with Crohn's disease. Dis Colon Rectum. 1993;36(9):840–3.
2. Bloom RJ, Larsen CP, Watt R, Oberhelman HA Jr. Complications and function of the continent ileostomy at the Cleveland clinic. World J Surg. 1988;12(2):148–54.
3. Wasmuth HH, Svinsas M, Trano G, et al. Surgical load and long-term outcome for patients with Kock continent ileostomy. Color Dis. 2007;9(8):713–7.
4. Kock NG. Intra-abdominal "reservoir" in patients with permanent ileostomy. Preliminary observations on a procedure resulting in fecal "continence" in five ileostomy patients. Arch Surg. 1969;99(2):223–31.
5. Borjesson L, Oresland T, Hulten L. The failed pelvic pouch: conversion to a continent ileostomy. Tech Coloproctol. 2004;8(2):102–5.
6. Kock NG, Myrvold HE, Nilsson LO, Philipson BM. Continent ileostomy. An account of 314 patients. Acta Chir Scand. 1981;147:67–72.
7. Nessar G, Wu JS. Evolution of continent ileostomy. World J Gastroenterol. 2012;18(27):3479–82.
8. Wasmuth HH, Myrvold HE. Durability of ileal pouch-anal anastomosis and continent ileostomy. Dis Colon Rectum. 2009;52(7):1285–9.
9. Aytac E, Ashburn J, Dietz DW. Is there still a role for continent ileostomy in the surgical treatment of inflammatory bowel disease? Inflamm Bowel Dis. 2014;20(12):2519–25.
10. Lepistö AH, Järvinen HJ. Durability of Kock continent ileostomy. Dis Colon Rectum. 2003;46(7):925–8.
11. Heuschen UA, Hinz U, Allemeyer EH, Autschbach F, Stern J, Lucas M, Herfarth C, Heuschen G. Risk factors for ileoanal J pouch-related septic complications in ulcerative colitis and familial adenomatous polyposis. Ann Surg. 2002;235(2):207–16.
12. Schluender SJ, Ippoliti A, Dubinsky M, Vasiliauskas EA, Papadakis KA, Mei L, Targan SR, Fleshner PR. Does infliximab influence surgical morbidity of ileal pouch-anal anastomosis in patients with ulcerative colitis? Dis Colon Rectum. 2007;50(11):1747–53.
13. Bauer JJ, Gorfine SR, Gelernt IM, Harris MT, Kreel I. Restorative proctocolectomy in patients older than fifty years. Dis Colon Rectum. 1997;40(5):562–5.
14. Mathis KL, Benavente-Chenhalls LA, Dozois EJ, Wolff BG, Larson DW. Short- and long-term surgical outcomes in patients undergoing proctocolectomy with ileal pouch-anal anastomosis in the setting of primary sclerosing cholangitis. Dis Colon Rectum. 2011;54(7):787–92.
15. Gu J, Stocchi L, Remzi F, Kiran RP. Factors associated with postoperative morbidity, reoperation and readmission rates after laparoscopic total abdominal colectomy for ulcerative colitis. Color Dis. 2013;15:1123–9.
16. Markel TA, Lou DC, Pfefferkorn M, Scherer K, West LR, Rouse T, et al. Steroids and poor nutrition are associated with infectious wound complications in children undergoing first stage procedures for ulcerative colitis. Surgery. 2008;144:540–5455–7.
17. Aberra FN, Lewis JD, Hass D, Rombeau JL, Osborne B, Lichtenstein GR. Corticosteroids and immunomodulators: postoperative infectious complication risk in inflammatory bowel disease patients. Gastroenterology. 2003;125:320–7.
18. Miki C, Ohmori Y, Yoshiyama S, Toiyama Y, Araki T, Uchida K, et al. Factors predicting postoperative infectious complications and early induction of inflammatory mediators in ulcerative colitis patients. World J Surg. 2007;31:522–52930–1.
19. Ferrante M, D'Hoore A, Vermeire S, Declerck S, Noman M, Van Assche G, et al. Corticosteroids but not infliximab increase short-term postoperative infectious complications in patients with ulcerative colitis. Inflamm Bowel Dis. 2009;15:1062–70.
20. Selvasekar CR, Cima RR, Larson DW, Dozois EJ, Harrington JR, Harmsen WS, et al. Effect of infliximab on short-term complications in patients undergoing operation for chronic ulcerative colitis. J Am Coll Surg. 2007;204:956–96262–3.
21. Mor IJ, Vogel JD, da Luz Moreira A, Shen B, Hammel J, Remzi FH. Infliximab in ulcerative colitis is associated with an increased risk of postoperative complications after restorative proctocolectomy. Dis Colon Rectum. 2008;51:1202–12077–10.

22. Norgard BM, Nielsen J, Qvist N, Gradel KO, de Muckadell OB, Kjeldsen J. Pre-operative use of anti-TNF-alpha agents and the risk of post-operative complications in patients with Crohn's disease – a nationwide cohort study. Aliment Pharmacol Ther. 2013;37:214–24.
23. Bregnbak D, Mortensen C, Bendtsen F. Infliximab and complications after colectomy in patients with ulcerative colitis. J Crohns Colitis. 2012;6:281–6.
24. Yang Z, Wu Q, Wang F, Wu K, Fan D. Meta-analysis: effect of preoperative infliximab use on early postoperative complications in patients with ulcerative colitis undergoing abdominal surgery. Aliment Pharmacol Ther. 2012;36:922–92.

Chapter 4
Patient Information

Christina Schulz and Rune Sjödahl

The purpose of this chapter is to summarize what doctors and other care providers should be aware of when giving information to patients before and after the construction of a continent ileostomy. Information given directly to the patient is usually based on a local pamphlet with more everyday language.

4.1 Various Scenarios the Surgeon Should Be Aware of When the Patient Is Informed Before Operation with a Continent Ileostomy/Kock Pouch

Conversion of a conventional ileostomy These patients have often difficulties to accept their stoma and are very much focused on the advantages with a continent ileostomy. It is very important for the surgeon to elucidate possible complications – both surgical and non-surgical. Dysmotility of the small bowel may imply that more frequent evacuations of the pouch are required than in the normal case.

Conversion of a pelvic pouch When the indication is organic complications one can expect a satisfying result. However, when there are functional disorders with frequent imperative emptyings, the bowel will probably have the same habits after the construction of a continent ileostomy. Pouchitis are easier to manage in a Kock pouch as continuous drainage is often effective within a week.

C. Schulz (✉)
Department of Surgery, University Hospital, Linköping, Sweden
e-mail: Christina.Schulz@regionostergotland.se

R. Sjödahl
Department of Clinical and Experimental Medicine, Linköping University, Linköping, Sweden
e-mail: Rune.Sjodahl@regionostergotland.se

© Springer Nature Switzerland AG 2019
P. Myrelid, M. Block (eds.), *The Kock Pouch*,
https://doi.org/10.1007/978-3-319-95591-9_4

Proctocolectomy with a primary continent ileostomy It is still a stoma that is a new situation for the patient. The small bowel function is important to analyse. The conversion to a conventional ileostomy is an option if the patient is not satisfied with the function.

Patients with Crohn's disease The risk is increased for chronic pouchitis and other complications. Maintenance treatment with immune-modulators could be offered from the beginning.

Patients with polyposis or cancer in the colon There are prerequisites for a good function when there are no signs of gastrointestinal dysmotility.

4.2   Information to Patients Before Construction of a Continent Ileostomy (Kock Pouch/Reservoir)

Description of a continent ileostomy A continent ileostomy means that the intestinal content is not emptied spontaneously from the small bowel as in patients with a conventional end-ileostomy. A one-way nipple valve and a pouch obtain the continence function. The operation has got its name – the Kock pouch – from the surgeon who invented the operation, Nils G Kock (Fig. 4.1).

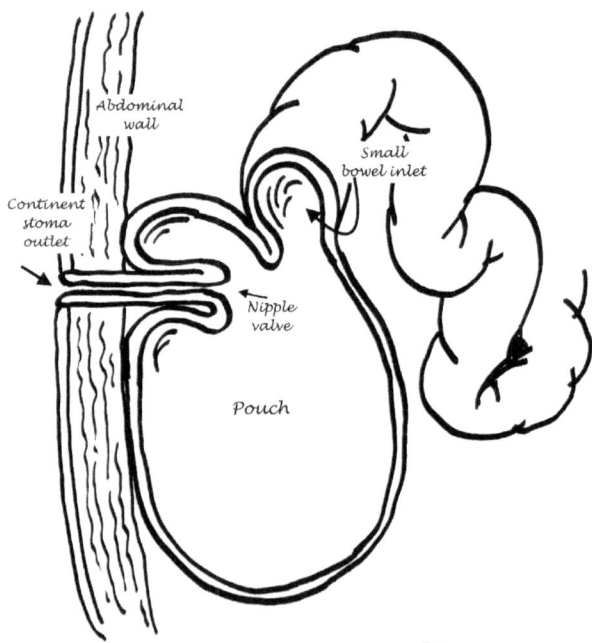

Fig 4.1 A simplified drawing of a Kock pouch describing the inlet, pouch, nipple and outlet

The intestinal content must be emptied with a rather thick catheter, which is introduced into the pouch through the flat ileostomy located at the right lower quadrant of the abdominal wall usually below the site for a conventional end-ileostomy.

Operation As in most other abdominal operations premedication and an epidural anaesthesia are used as well as general anaesthesia. About half a meter of the lowest part of the small bowel is used to construct the pouch and the nipple valve. The ileostomy is sewn flat with the skin. A thick catheter is placed through the stoma into the pouch, sutured to the abdominal wall, and connected to a bag for sampling of the intestinal content. The first hours or sometimes overnight are spent in the postoperative ward before transportation to the surgical ward. Rarely a deviating loop ileostomy is used with the aim to protect the pouch.

Postoperative care After the operation fluid and sometimes nutrition is given intravenously until the stomach and bowel is functioning and the patient can drink and eat. The diet should be light and it is necessary to chew the food very thoroughly as the waste must come through the draining catheter. It is wise to avoid for instance fibre, mushrooms and nuts as these may block the catheter. In order to avoid overload and distension of the pouch and to facilitate healing, the pouch is drained continuously with a thick ileostomy catheter during the first weeks. The ileostomy catheter is sutured to the skin during operation, or postoperatively sometimes fixed with adhesive plaster to the skin and as mentioned before connected to a tube draining into a bag. All that is covered with a bandage, which is changed when there has been leakage or after shower. Obviously this arrangement can be experienced as bulky and perceived as a barrier to daily life but it should be stressed how important it is for an optimal healing. The pouch is washed with water 2–4 times a day during 4 weeks. After 2 weeks the ileostomy catheter is closed intermittently so to increase the volume of the pouch. The stay in hospital is usually 1–2 weeks and the time for being out of work is often 6–8 weeks. In the case of a protecting loop ileostomy it is usually closed after 2–3 months and then the dilatation of the pouch starts.

Normal function Every day up to one litre of bowel content and as much flatus is produced. Most persons empty their pouches 3–5 times a day but not during night. Some patients have a feeling of pressure when it is time to empty the pouch. The pouch should not be overloaded as it may cause some trouble for the catheter to pass through the nipple. Between the evacuations of the pouch there are no leakage of gas or bowel content. The time to empty the pouch is about 5 min and then the stoma is cleaned with toilet tissue and protected with an absorbing dressing.

Advantages with a continent ileostomy

- Full freedom for all common activities, including sex life
- Flush low stoma and no stoma bag
- No restrictions of clothes
- No smell

- Decide themselves the time for emptying
- Feeling of having an intact body and improved self confidence
- Good end result can be expected even after repeated reoperations provided the function of the small bowel is normal

Disadvantages with a continent ileostomy

- Dependence of an ileostomy catheter, i.e. it must always be accessible
- Dependence of a suitable place for emptying
- Recurrent pouchitis
- Secretion from the mucosa of the stoma requiring frequent change of dressing
- Surgical complications occur commonly (nipple dysfunction, stenosis of the stoma or the inlet to the pouch)

The patient should be offered to meet a man or a woman in the same age with a continent ileostomy to discuss various things as food habits, sports, and sex life. A pamphlet containing information about the continent ileostomy before and after the operation should be given to the patient.

The information is rather complex and therefore an informed consent might be of value. A proposal of a simple checklist for the patient and the surgeon is presented at the end of this chapter.

4.3   Information to Patients After Construction of a Continent Ileostomy

The stoma therapist usually gives this information and training but the patient is also stimulated to read the pamphlet on continent ileostomy by her- or himself. The patients should be aware that this is an uncommon operation and many doctors and nurses are not familiar with the function and various complications. It is important for the patient to know that during the time period with continuous drainage of the pouch certain activities like long travels should be avoided. For the rest of his or her life the patient must feel responsibility for taking care of the continent ileostomy and realize that like other intestinal stomas it does not live its own life without careful attention. It is not uncommon that the patients are disappointed the first time after the operation and may regret their decision. However, soon they become satisfied with their new life.

The ileostomy catheter is removed 4 weeks after the operation and the patient is trained to empty and wash the pouch. Initially the volume of the pouch is only 70–100 ml but after increasing the times of closure of the catheter the volume is gradually increased and soon reach 500 ml and even more.

Emptying of the pouch This can be done directly into the toilet when sitting on the edge of the lavatory. Otherwise the bowel content is collected in a bag that is closed and put into garbage.

Advice regarding food habits A general rule is that persons with a continent ileostomy should try to drink and eat without any restrictions but using common sense. Food like beans, peas, citrus fruits, asparagus, mushrooms, fruit skins and nuts should not be eaten in large amounts as they may block the passage through the catheter. If that happens the catheter is withdrawn and rinsed before it is reinserted. Solid bowel content is treated with increased intake of fluid. The pamphlet contains examples of food that may cause abdominal pain, increased amounts of flatus, and cause loose or solid bowel content.

Sexual life The change in the body image caused by a continent ileostomy can be both positive and negative depending on the individual starting point. It is not unusual with a decreased interest in sexual activity a various time after the operation but it is often temporary. It is important to ask the patient to talk about the feelings with her or his partner.

Travel Stoma equipment and salt tablets should be stored in more than one bag. If it is not advisable to drink the water also use non-sparkling mineral water o wash the pouch if necessary. Discussion with the stoma therapist or surgeon if any medication might be necessary (e.g. antibiotics, constipating agents) is advisable.

4.3.1 Non-Surgical Complications

Stomal flux This occurs less often than with a conventional ileostomy but is treated in the same way, i.e. with increased fluid intake, constipating agents and salt tablets.

Pouchitis Patients are informed that most common complication is one or two episodes of pouchitis. This is an inflammation of the pouch resulting in fever, abdominal pain, bloating and a need of emptying the pouch more frequently. Pouchitis will in most cases be cured with a course of antibiotics in a week or two. In recurrent pouchits other kinds of treatment may be added, such as anti-inflammatory agents or drainage during night-time or even continuously.

4.3.2 Surgical complications

It is important to stress that most surgical complications can be managed successfully with surgical corrections. Leakage of flatus or bowel content almost always is due to slippage of the valve. It can be cured with a revision of the nipple valve, or by construction of a new nipple. Fistulae can often be cured as well as a stenosis of the stoma.

Some reasons to contact the stoma therapist:

- Leakage of flatus or bowel content. It can indicate nipple dysfunction due to slipping of the valve or to pouchitis. Slipping of the valve is often associated with difficulties to pass the ileostomy catheter into the pouch. Colourless secretion is often due to secretion of mucus from the stomal mucosa.
- Prolapse of the nipple (looks like a conventional ileostomy)
- Fistulous opening to the peristomal skin
- An urge to empty and/or an increased frequency of emptying. This may indicate the presence of a pouchitis.
- Signs of gastroenteritis with production of substantially increased volume of bowel content during more than 1 day may require substitution with intravenous fluids. Persons without the absorption capacity of the colon are more sensitive to dehydration and kidney-failure.

The initial treatment by the stoma therapist is often an advice to let the ileostomy catheter remain in the pouch and if necessary connect it with a bag.

Situations when the emergency department of the hospital should be contacted

- Blocked passage through the catheter and no effect of changing position of the catheter or flushing of the catheter.
- The catheter cannot pass into the pouch
- Distended abdomen, colic pain and vomiting

4.4 Proposal to an informed consent

I have received information by a surgeon and a stoma therapist and understood the following about a continent ileostomy/Kock pouch

- The principles of the operation
- The postoperative care
- The normal function of a continent ileostomy
- The advantages and disadvantages of a continent ileostomy
- The risk of complications requiring reoperations
- The risk of pouchitis
- The risk of removing the pouch and getting a conventional stoma
- The possibility to contact a stoma therapist when necessary (name

  ....tel ....e-mail ....)

I understand that

- I can change my mind before admittance to hospital for the operation
- If it is best for me my doctor can change my treatment
- Doctors under training can participate in the treatment

- No guarantee can be given for a successful operation

Date ....
Name of the patient ....

4.5   Surgeon

I am responsible for giving information about the risks, the benefits and expected
result of the operation with a continent ileostomy (description of the operation using
a figure, anaesthesia, treatment of postoperative pain, wound treatment, early and
late complications, postoperative support and control), information about alternative treatments, and occupational groups who will participate in the treatment.

Name ....
....

Chapter 5
Kock Pouch Construction

Pär Myrelid and Mattias Block

5.1 Technique

At both centers we always have two experienced surgeons performing or revising Kock pouches, preferably accompanied by a third surgeon training to become an experienced Kock pouch surgeon as well.

After the previous Brooke ileostomy has been taken down (or a proctocolectomy or a completion proctectomy has been performed) the first step is to measure the amount of ileum needed for the creation of the pouch. A total amount of 45 cm of the last part of the ileum is used (Fig. 5.1). At every 15 cm a marking suture is made in order to not make a mistake later on. The next step is to make an approximately 30 cm long incision anti-mesenteric on the bowel (Fig. 5.2a, c), note the somewhat extended incision on the proximal end. This asymmetric incision is to make sure there is distance between the inlet of the pouch and the nipple valve when the pouch is finished. It is often easy to use the suction inside the bowel lumen when creating the long and straight incision (Fig. 5.2b).

After completing the incision the next step is to suture the back-wall of the pouch. This could be done with a running full through or seromuscular absorbable suture (Fig. 5.3a, b). The suture should be started in the most distal end of the incision joined to the proximal part of the same, but leaving the asymmetric proximal part of the incision until later. By starting at this end, and using a running suture, it will prevent the back wall from becoming wrinkled and uneven as the last part of the incision will smooth itself (Fig. 5.3c).

P. Myrelid (✉)
Linköping University Hospital, Department of Surgery, Linköping University, Department of Clinical and Experimental Medicine, Linköping, Sweden
e-mail: par.myrelid@liu.se

M. Block
Department of Surgery, Colorectal Unit, Sahlgrenska University Hospital/Östra, Gothenburg, Sweden

© Springer Nature Switzerland AG 2019
P. Myrelid, M. Block (eds.), *The Kock Pouch*,
https://doi.org/10.1007/978-3-319-95591-9_5

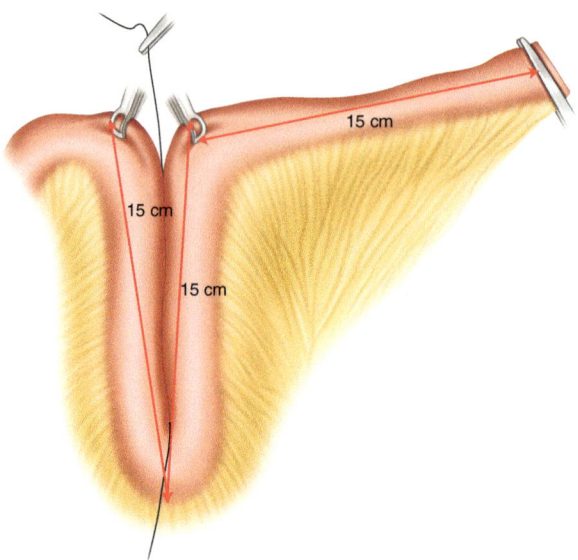

Fig. 5.1 Sutures are made to mark every 15 cm (of the first 45 cm) of the distal ileum

The peritoneum of the mesentery is then removed triangularly on both sides on the proximal two thirds of the outlet from the pouch using scissors and/or diathermy (Fig. 5.4). The base of the triangle should be at the bowel wall and the tip towards the mesenteric root. In patients with a more thickened mesentery parts of the fat may need to be excised as well in order to make it possible to intussuscept the efferent limb of the ileum and creating the nipple valve.

The nipple valve is initially made by making an intussusception of the efferent limb using a Babcock clamp. A firm grip is made in the bowel wall and then carefully completing the intussusception (Fig. 5.5a, b). When the nipple has a good length of at least 4–5 cm the stapling device is used, which usually makes the nipple somewhat longer reaching the goal of 5–6 cm. The stapling is made by using a knife-less GIA 60 mm, TA 60 mm or similar (Fig. 5.6a, b). A minimum of three firings are made and with meticulous care not firing into the mesentery. One firing should be made at each side of the mesentery (which is most often both visible and palpable as a thickening of the nipple) and then a third firing at the ante-mesenteric side (Fig. 5.6a). In some cases a fourth firing can be made. If using a TA device or similar there will be a hole after the pin of the instrument at the base of the nipple, and this needs to be closed with a stich. At this time the nipple is quite stiff and bluish in its colour but it will recover.

The last part of making the pouch itself is the closure of the anterior wall of the pouch. Once again a running absorbable suture is used in a seromuscular manner. Starting at the mid of the pouch one running suture is made proximally and a second distally on the previous incision (Fig. 5.7). When doing this one has to make sure the asymmetry of the incision is kept as this will create a distance

Fig. 5.2 (**a**) A 30 cm long anti-mesenteric incision is made on the distal ileum and this incision is often extended past the proximal marking suture. (**b**) The cover to the suction is inserted into the bowel lumen to simplify the long incision of the distal ileum. (**c**) The difference in the length of the incision from (**a**) seen in a per-operative photography as well

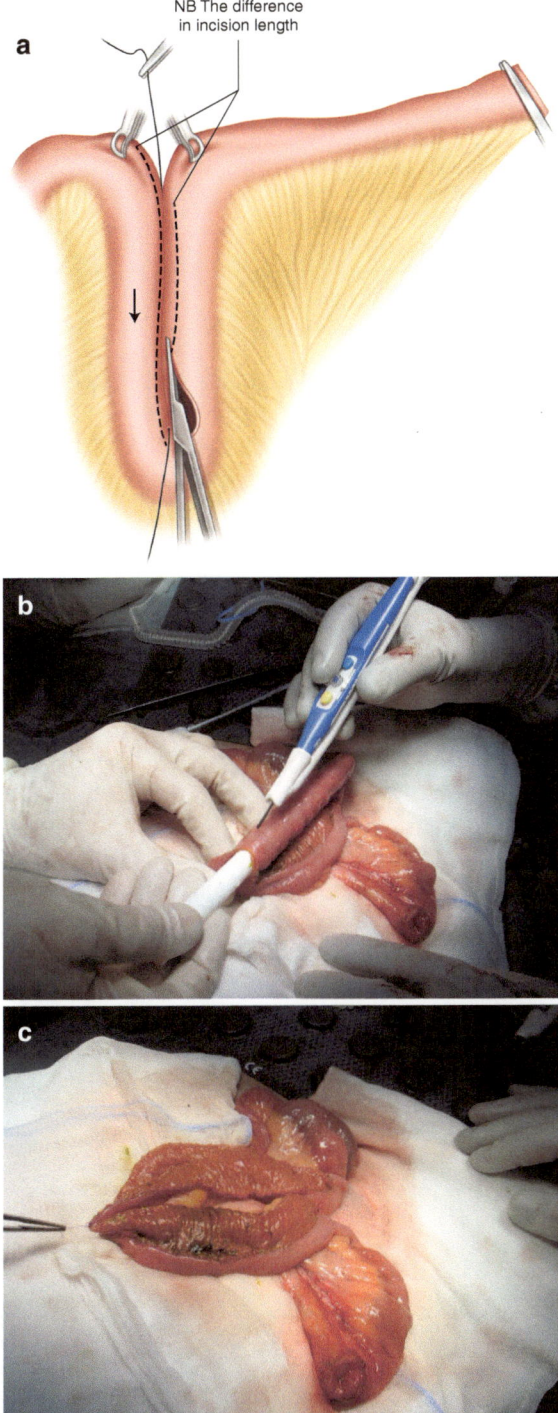

Fig. 5.3 (**a**) The back wall of the pouch is sutured with a running suture starting with joining the proximal and distal ends of the incision, but leaving the asymmetric proximal part of the incision. (**b**) The back wall of the pouch is sutured, starting from the proximal and distal ends of the incision, which will make sure the back wall suture will not become frilly. (**c**) The back wall of the pouch is completed

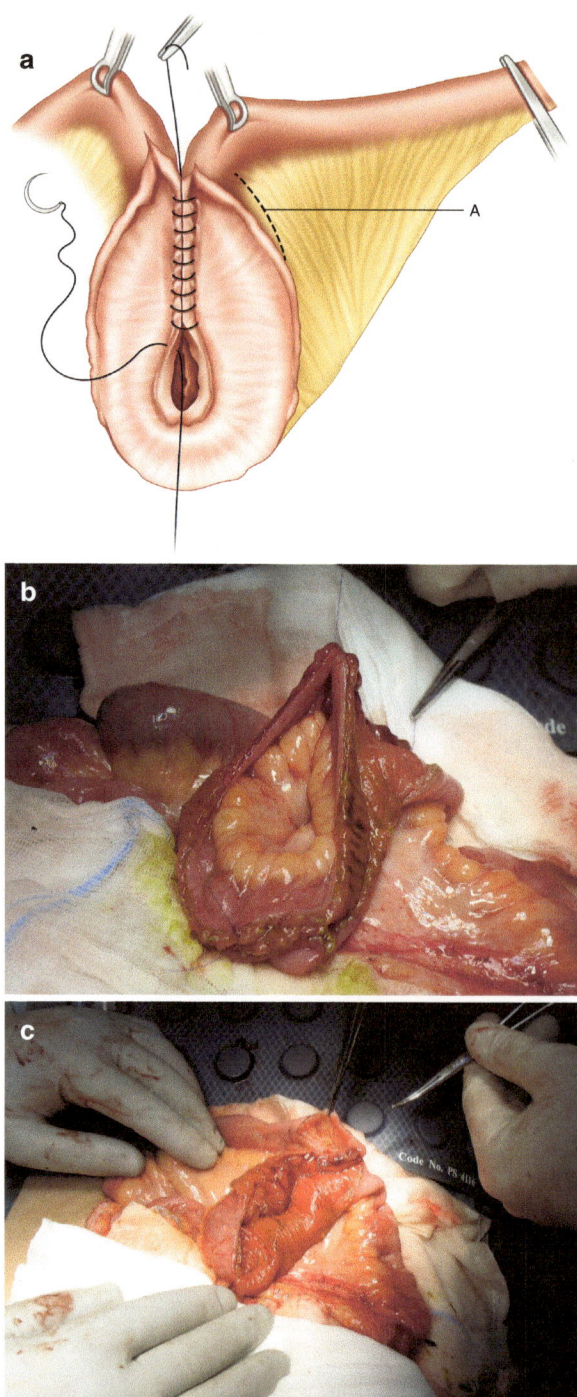

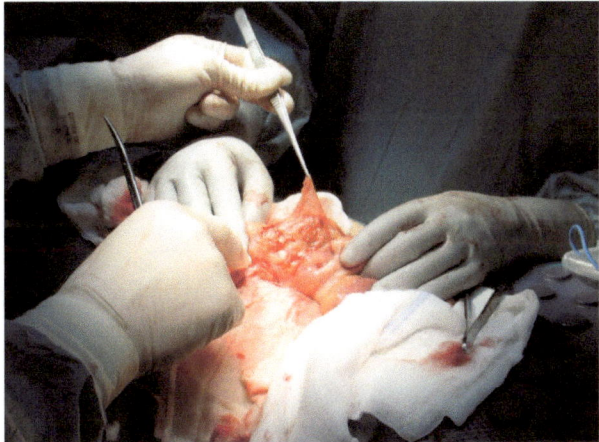

Fig. 5.4 The peritoneum of the mesentery is removed triangularly on both sides on the proximal 2/3 of the outlet from the pouch; which will become the nipple valve

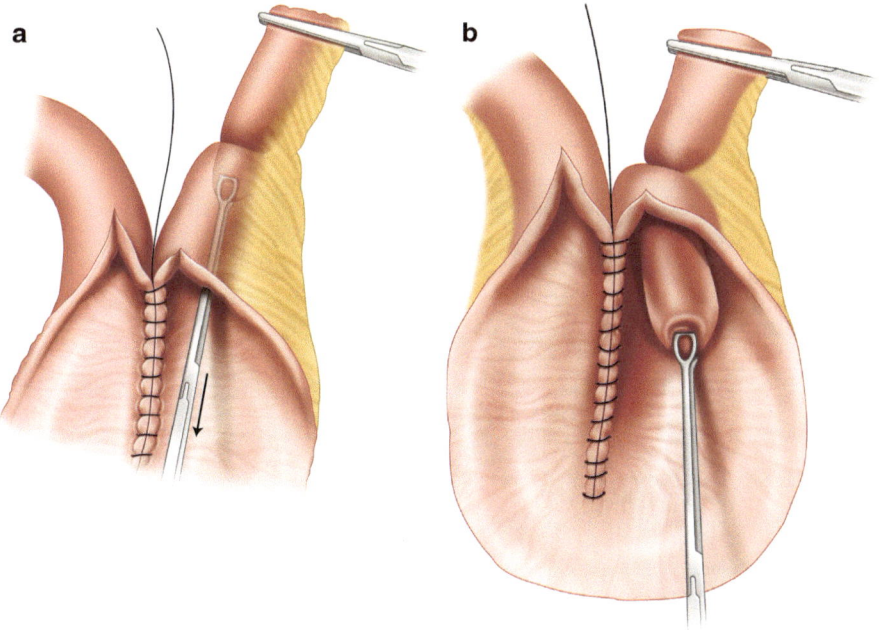

Fig. 5.5 (**a**) First part of the intussusception of the nipple valve using Babcocks. The peritoneum is removed from both sides of the mesentery before the intussusception manoeuvre of the nipple. (**b**) Second step in creation of the nipple valve. The nipple valve should be approximately 5–6 cm long when finished

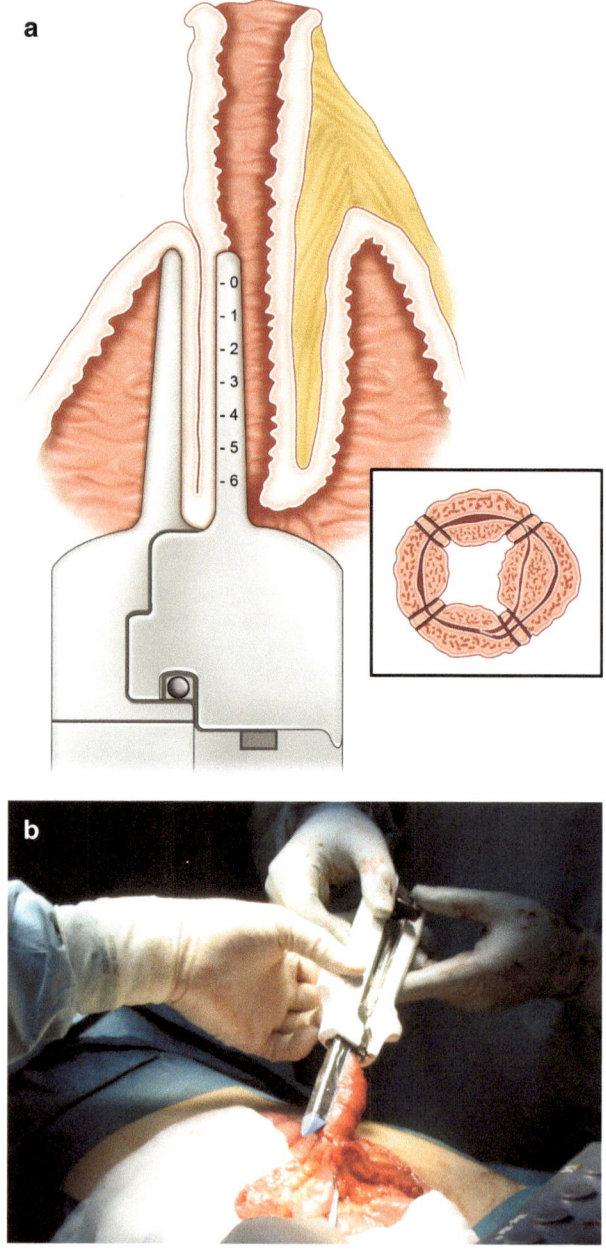

Fig. 5.6 (**a**) Staple fixation of the nipple valve using a knife-less GIA 60 mm, TA 60 mm or similar. When using a TA instrument there will be a puncturing at the nipple base after each firing that needs to be over-sewn. (**b**) Stapling of the nipple using a knife-less GIA 60 mm

Fig. 5.7 Closure of the anterior wall of the pouch. When doing this you need to make sure the distance between the inlet and the nipple valve is enough, and this is made by maintaining the asymmetry of the incision of the inlet part

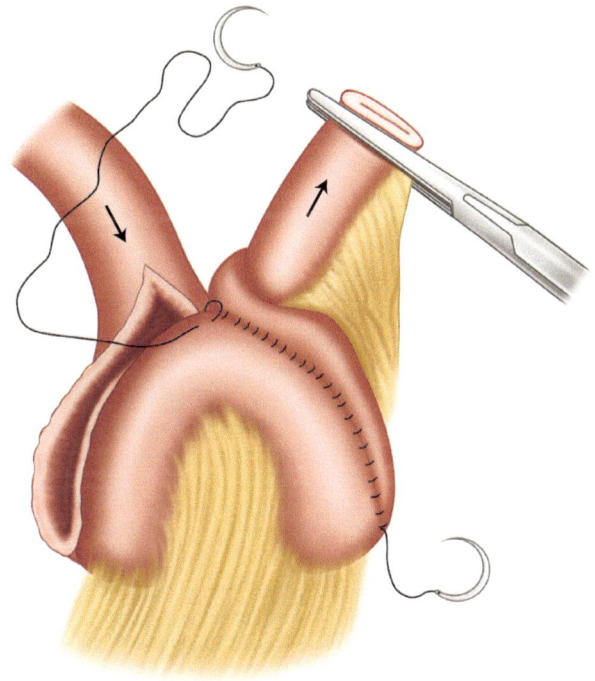

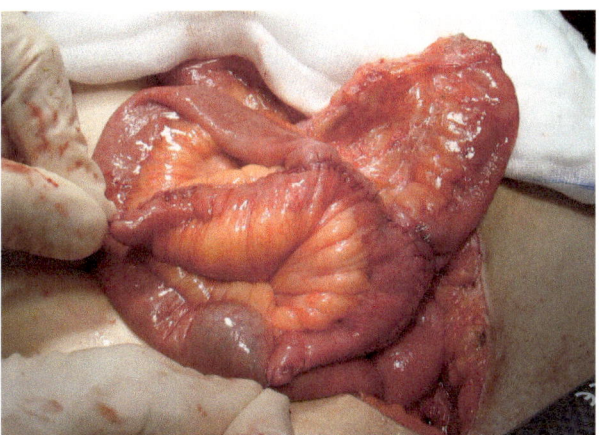

Fig. 5.8 The suturing of the pouch is almost finished and the last step is to create the base of the nipple valve by interrupted sutures between the outlet of the nipple and the body of the pouch

between the inlet of the pouch and the nipple valve at the final stage (Fig. 5.7). The last part of the suturing of the pouch itself is to make the base of the nipple by interrupted resorbable sutures between the proximal part of the outlet and the body of the pouch (Fig. 5.8).

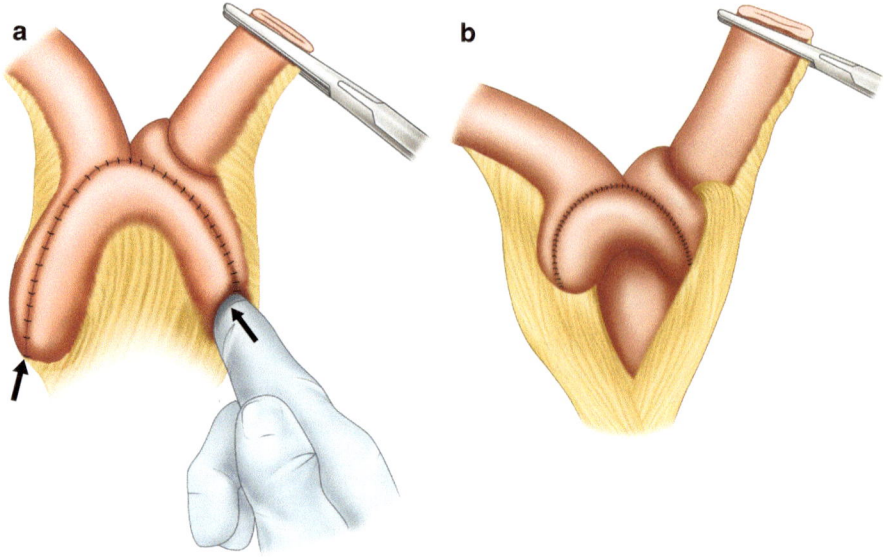

Fig. 5.9 (**a**) The both ends of the banana shaped Kock pouch are pushed through the mesentery. (**b**) The both ends of the banana shaped Kock pouch are pushed through the mesentery

The following step is one of the most difficult parts to describe in the creation of a Kock pouch. When the suturing of the pouch is completed it will somewhat like a small banana (Figs. 5.7 and 5.8). The both ends of the banana shaped pouch should then be pushed through the mesentery (Fig. 5.9a). When the both ends are pushed through the whole way a rather spherical pouch has been created, one of the Hallmarks of the Kock pouch (Figs 5.9a, b).

At this stage a first test of the continence is made by inserting the Medina catheter through the nipple valve into the pouch. The assistant gently compresses the inlet with his/her fingers while the surgeon uses an air-filled syringe to gently fill the pouch with air. To make sure the air is not leaking in between the fillings the catheter should be clamped and opened only when inserting air. When the pouch is filled the catheter is removed (still clamped) and it should then be continent (Fig. 5.10). If so, the Medina catheter is once again inserted and the air is evacuated.

If the patient has had an ileostomy before this could be reused but quite often the patients prefer a lower stoma opening below the waist line. When doing a new stoma opening one should keep it more narrow than a standard ileostomy, but wide enough to contain both the efferent limb of the bowel and a Medina catheter at the same time. After completing the stoma opening it is time to suture the pouch to the abdominal wall. The weakest part will be at the level of the mesentery as the cuff of the nipple base is non-existing here. In order to diminish the risk of detachment of the pouch from the abdominal wall later on one should try to make two

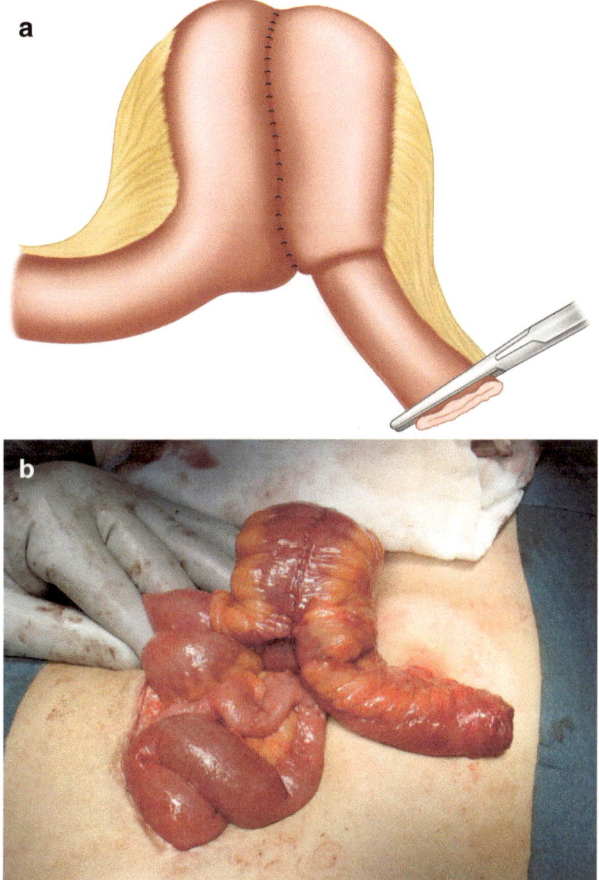

Fig. 5.10 (**a**) When the both ends are pushed through the mesentery a rather spherical pouch has been created. (**b**) When the both ends are pushed through the mesentery a rather spherical pouch has been created with the inlet to the left and the outlet and nipple valve to the right

sutures in the anterior sheath laterally in the stoma opening; most easily made from the outside of the abdominal wall and with the sutures later brought to the inside of the abdominal cavity (Fig. 5.11). These sutures are then secured (but yet not tied) in close proximity to the mesentery on the base of the pouch. Some units prefer slowly resorbable sutures while others prefer non-absorbable sutures. After the initial two sutures at least six more sutures are secured in the cuff at the base of the nipple and to the posterior sheath of the rectus muscle. When all eight sutures are in place they are tied one by one, starting in a lateral to medial way, making sure none of the sutures are crossed. When all the sutures are tied the pouch is secured to the abdominal wall (Fig. 5.12) and a second test of continence is made in the same manner as described above.

Fig. 5.11 Two anchoring stiches are made laterally through the anterior sheath of the rectus muscle. These stiches are then inserted to the abdominal cavity and secured to the cuff of the nipple base as close to the mesenteric fold as possible

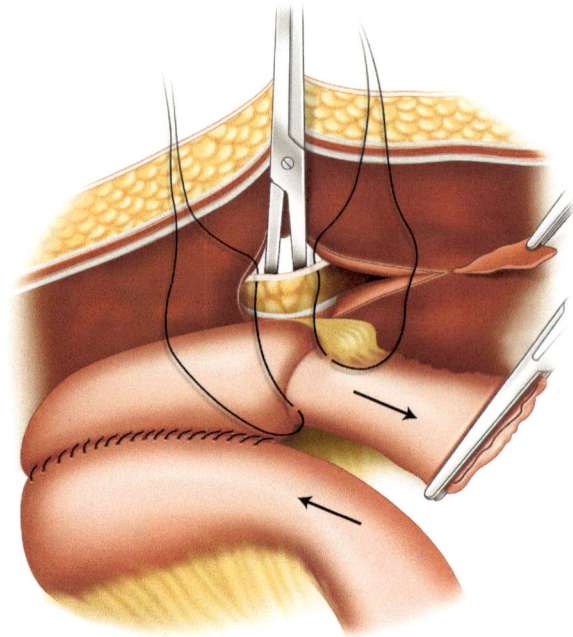

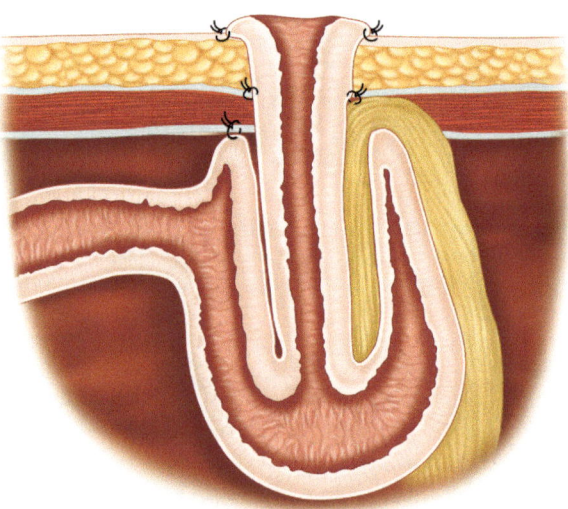

Fig. 5.12 A total number of eight sutures should be made around the base of the nipple valve. At least two of them should be to the anterior sheath of the rectus muscle (laterally) while the remaining six could be between the cuff of the pouch and the posterior sheath of the rectus muscle

If the pouch is easily intubated and the pouch is continent it is time to trim the stoma. Any redundant ileum of the efferent limb is excised at or just above the skin level and interrupted sutures are made between the skin and bowel wall. It is always easier to remove a little bit of extra small bowel later on while a too short efferent limb might cause a major revision including the need of a rotation of the pouch and creation of a new nipple.

Before closing the abdomen the Medina catheter is positioned with its tip passing through the opening of the nipple valve but without putting any pressure on the bottom of the pouch, as this could cause a necrotic wound and perforation later on. One way to make sure the catheter is kept in the right position is to tie a knot around it securely at the level of the skin. This can later be used as a mark ta make sure the catheter is not pushed in too far or pulled out too much. The catheter is then secured with sutures and tape as described in Chaps. 9 and 11.

Chapter 6
Kock Pouch Construction: Our Approach

Mantaj S. Brar, Anthony de Buck Van Overstraeten, Michael Corrin, Robin McLeod, and Zane Cohen

6.1 Introduction

Following the innovative description of the Continent Ileostomy by Professor Nils G Kock in 1969 many modifications have been attempted to improve patient outcomes. Based on the tutelage of Professor Kock, extensive collaboration with our colleagues in Gothenburg, and our personal experience over more than four decades, we will briefly discuss the evolution of the procedure and describe our current approach to the creation of a Kock pouch. However, it is important to note that the creation of the Kock pouch may require individualized decisions related to the thickness of the mesentery, the thickness of the abdominal wall, and previous surgery on the terminal ileum.

On review of our experience at Mount Sinai Hospital, between 1976 and 2013, our institution has created and/or revised Kock pouches of 194 patients. Over this time period, our approach to the procedure has evolved. Primarily we have employed a 3-limb Kock pouch (S-shaped) given the increased capacity of the pouch to allow for easier manipulation of the valve; however, approximately 20% of pouches in the late 1980s and 1990s were 2-limb pouches (K-shaped) as originally described. Given the concerns with valve slippage, various techniques have been employed to stabilize the valve within the pouch. A fascial sling around the neck of the valve to reinforce the valve mechanism was employed early in our experience in the 1970s, and was replaced by a polypropylene mesh sling as our preferred approach in the 1980s and 1990s; however, this has since been abandoned due to mesh erosions and

M. S. Brar (✉) · A. de Buck Van Overstraeten · R. McLeod · Z. Cohen
Mount Sinai Hospital, Zane Cohen Centre for Digestive Diseases, Department of Surgery,
University of Toronto, Toronto, ON, Canada
e-mail: Mantaj.Brar@sinaihealthsystem.ca

M. Corrin
Biomedical Communications Graduate Program, Department of Biology,
University of Toronto, Toronto, ON, Canada

© Springer Nature Switzerland AG 2019
P. Myrelid, M. Block (eds.), *The Kock Pouch*,
https://doi.org/10.1007/978-3-319-95591-9_6

fistulas. Since the early 1980s, nearly all valves have been secured with a stapled technique. In addition, we now routinely staple the valve to the pouch anteriorly with extension of the staple line on to the efferent limb (outlet). Lastly, for revisions due to valve slippage, we have been performing a fundoplication of the efferent limb by wrapping and suturing the distal pouch around the base of the efferent limb.

With a mean follow-up of 27 years, 70% of our patients continue to have a functioning Kock pouch (estimated 20-year pouch survival of 67%), and report an excellent quality of life with 80–90% reporting minimal or no restrictions to their personal and professional lives. The most common pouch complication was valve slippage (40%) which occurred both early and late (from 2 months to 26 years). All patients underwent surgical revision after valve slippage with 40% having no further slippage and 60% requiring subsequent revision or excision of the pouch. Other complications of the pouch requiring surgical revision included fistula formation (19%), outlet stenosis (14%), and valve prolapse (11%). No patients in this cohort developed dysplasia or malignancy of the pouch, and the cumulative risk of pouchitis was 30%. Retrospectively, it is difficult to conclusively attribute the technical modifications of the procedure to outcomes given the modest sample sizes for each modification and the limits of controlling for confounders. Based on our experience we feel the current approach described here affords a selected group of highly motivated patients robust continent pouch function that is acceptable in light of the perioperative complications and risk of revisional surgery.

6.2   Technique

Prior to presentation to the operating theatre, the patient's abdomen should be marked at the preferred site for the continent ileostomy stoma. This should be done by an experienced enteral stoma nurse given the more caudal positioning of the stoma than conventional ileostomy. The site should be just above the pubic hair line on the right side and through the rectus muscle. The patient is placed in supine position if an end-ileostomy is present, or in lithotomy position if a proctectomy or proctocolectomy is performed during the same operation. A lower midline incision is made, the terminal ileum is mobilized (either the ileostomy is fully mobilized, or the terminal ileum is divided at the ileocecal valve if a proctocolectomy is being performed simultaneously), and approximately 60–70 cm of ileum are freed from adhesions and exteriorized. The abdominal cavity is protected with surgical towels to minimize contamination.

With the use of Babcocks, the terminal ileum is oriented to construct the pouch. The terminal 15 cm is left for the efferent limb and the nipple valve, but in the patient with a thick abdominal wall this may need to be longer (better too long than too short, as the efferent limb is drawn through the abdominal wall only after the whole pouch is created). Three limbs of 10–12 cm are arranged to form an S-pouch using Babcock tissue clamps. A running suture in the seromuscular layer is placed for the outer layer of the anastomosis between each of the limbs (Fig. 6.1). A non-crushing bowel clamp is applied to the small bowel proximal to the pouch and an

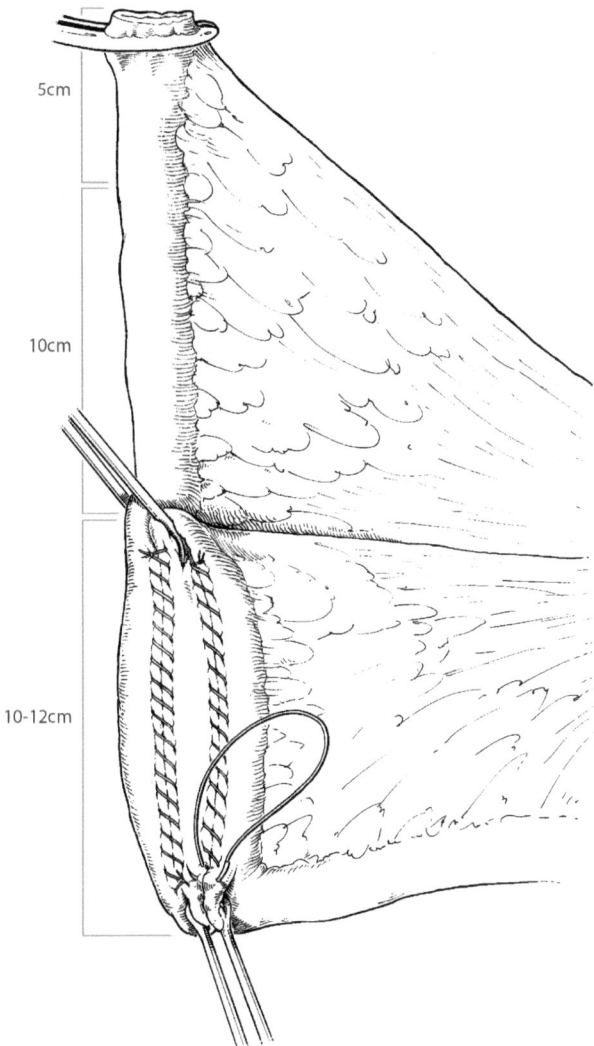

Fig. 6.1 Orientation of the terminal ileum for pouch construction with suture of the back wall of the pouch

anti-mesenteric enterotomy is made through all three limbs (Fig. 6.2). A running suture in a full-thickness fashion is placed for the inner layer of the anastomosis starting at the apices of the limbs, leaving 2 cm of length at the two apices to allow for later closure of the anterior layer of the pouch (Fig. 6.3). To allow for intussusception of the nipple valve and to facilitate adhesion formation, a triangular area of mesentery adjacent to the bowel used for the nipple valve is deperitonealized and redundant fat is removed from the mesentery using diathermy and/or scissors on both sides while preserving the blood supply (Fig. 6.4). Using Babcock clamps, the efferent limb is then intussuscepted into the pouch to create a 5–7 cm nipple valve

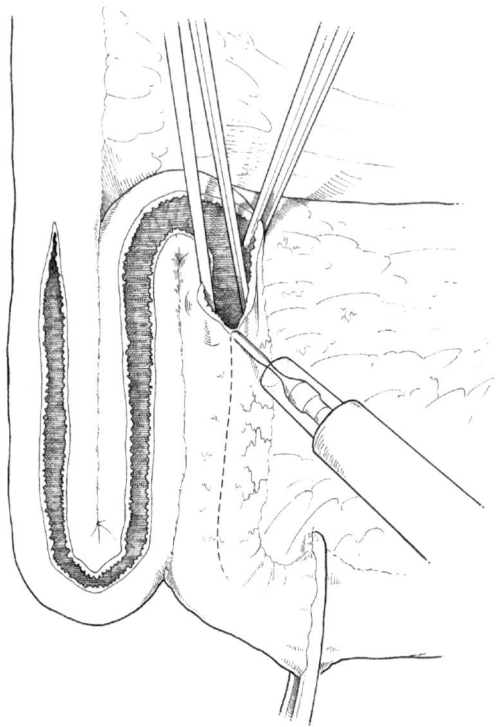

Fig. 6.2 The anterior wall of the pouch is incised with cautery

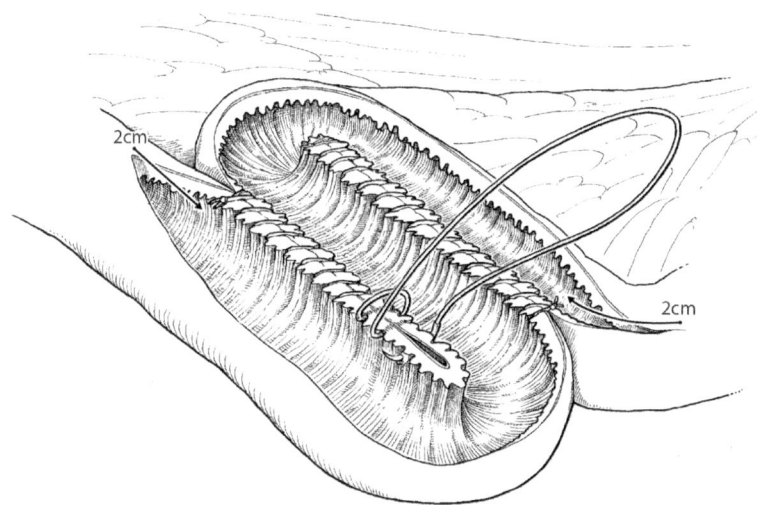

Fig. 6.3 The second layer of the back wall is sutured using two running sutures, leaving 2 cm of length on either end of the pouch wall free

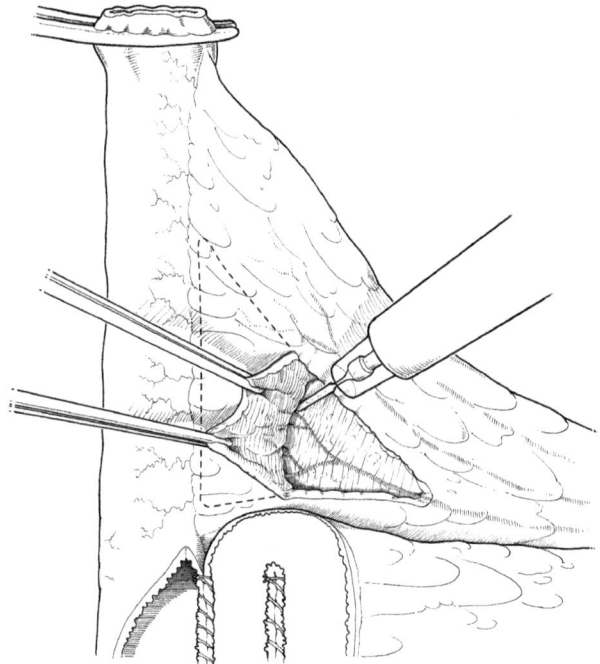

Fig. 6.4 De-fatting the mesentery to the nipple valve

(Fig. 6.5). We employ a stapled nipple fixation, starting with the use of a knife-less GIA 60 mm stapler applied 2 times at approximately 4 and 8 o'clock radially to avoid injury to the mesentery which is centered at 6 o'clock (Fig. 6.6). Once the posterior nipple valve is secured, the anterior wall of the pouch is partially closed using a running suture starting at the distal aspect of the pouch and continuing to just beyond the nipple valve (Fig. 6.7). The most proximal staples in each row of the TLH 90 stapler are then removed to preserve the blood supply to the nipple and to leave a portion of the anterior wall of the pouch free to be closed afterward. The nipple valve is then secured anteriorly to the anterior wall of the pouch by firing the TLH 90 stapler twice at 10 and 2 o'clock, extending the staple line to the efferent limb distal to the nipple (Fig. 6.8). This results in a small puncture in the efferent limb at the site of the stapler pin that requires a purse-string stitch for closure. It is common that the nipple will appear somewhat dusky after firing the securing staplers, but we have not had any early nipple necrosis; the surgeon should not wait for improvement in the appearance of the nipple prior to closing the pouch. The remainder of the anterior wall of the pouch is then closed using a running suture (Fig. 6.9). We then perform a test of the nipple valve mechanism; this is performed by placing a bowel clamp on the afferent limb, inserting the Medina® catheter into the pouch, insufflating the pouch with air using a bulb syringe attached to a Medina® catheter while placing a clamp on the catheter to prevent evacuation of air in between repeated syringe insufflations; we then remove the Medina® catheter to ensure the

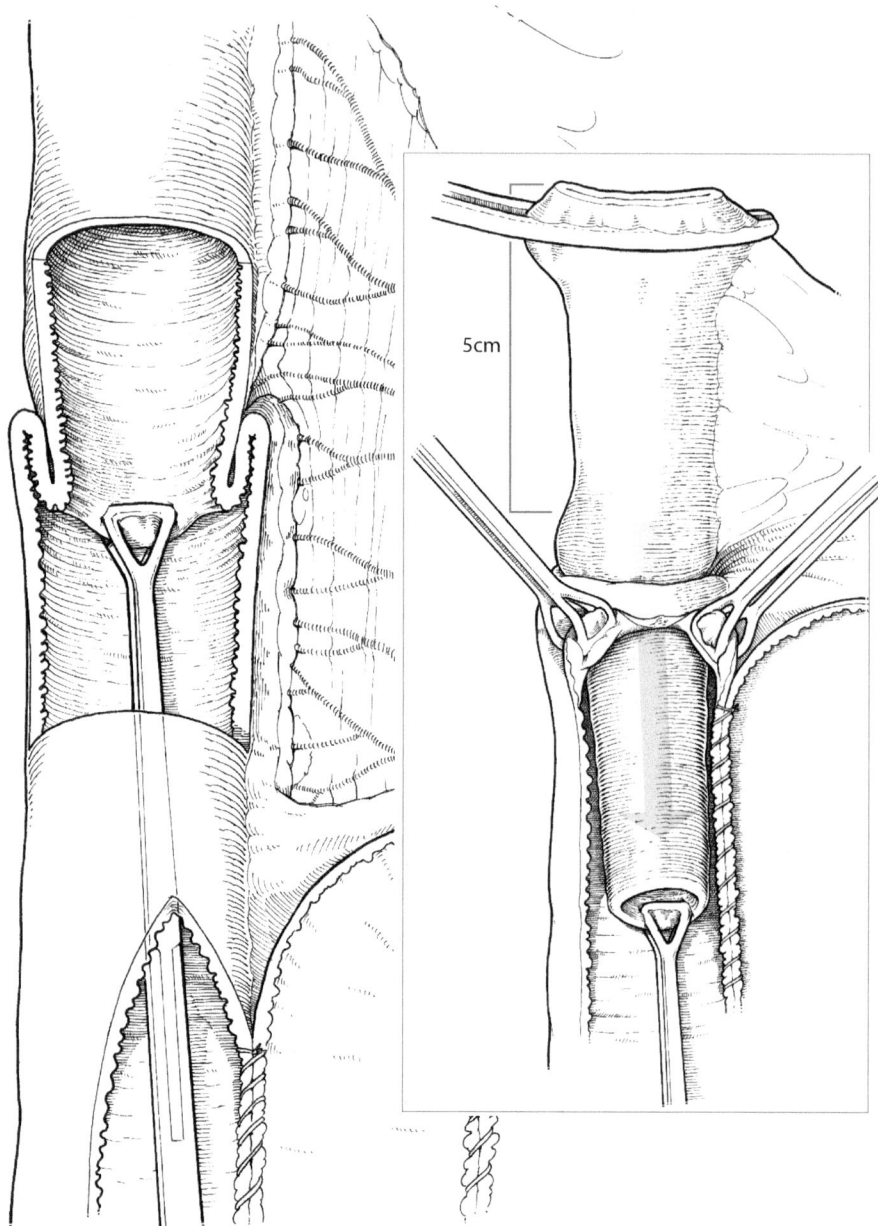

5cm

Fig. 6.5 Intussusception of the nipple valve using Babcocks

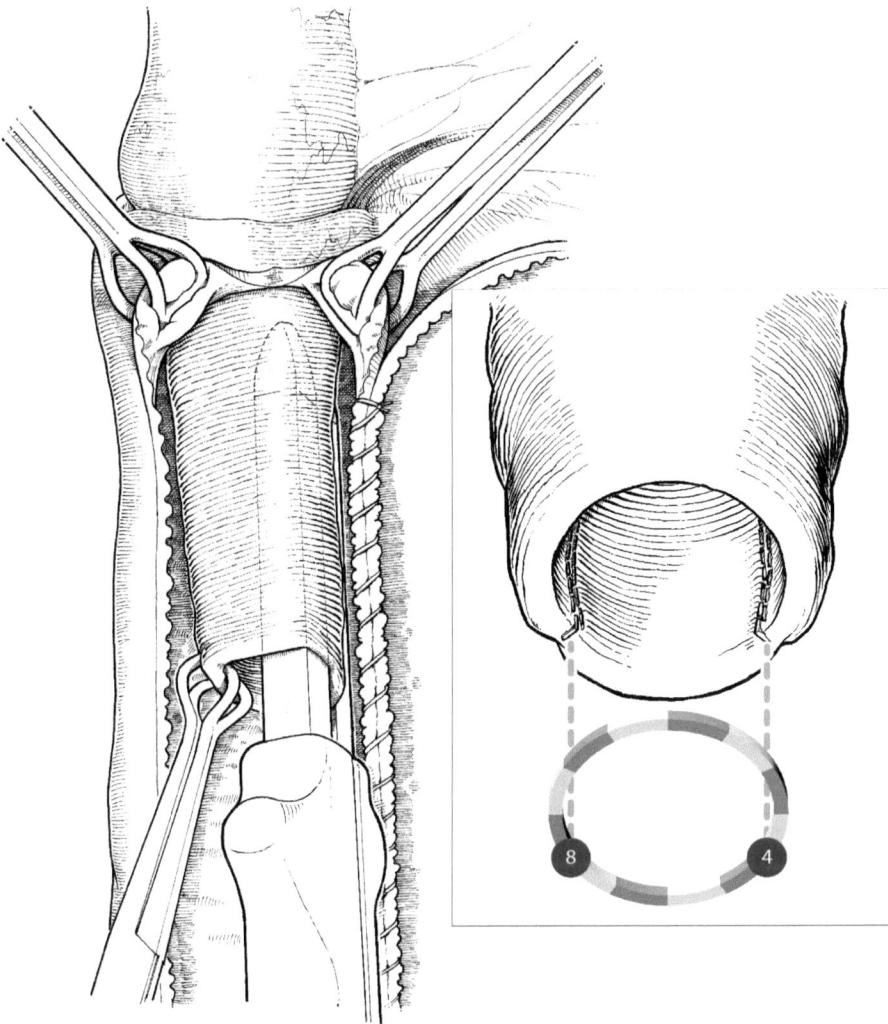

Fig. 6.6 Posterior staple fixation of the nipple valve at 4 and 8 o'clock using a knifeless GIA stapler

valve is competent. Once the test is satisfactory, the cuff of the pouch is secured radially to the efferent limb (outlet) using interrupted sutures (Fig. 6.10).

Once the pouch is constructed and continence has been confirmed, the pouch is positioned ideally in the right lower abdomen so that the inferior portion sits on, and

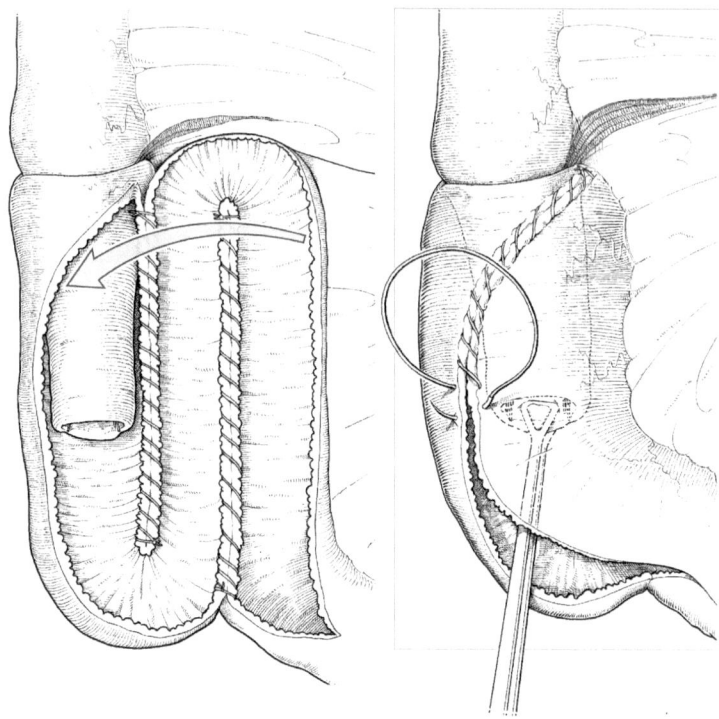

Fig. 6.7 Partial closure of the anterior wall of the pouch

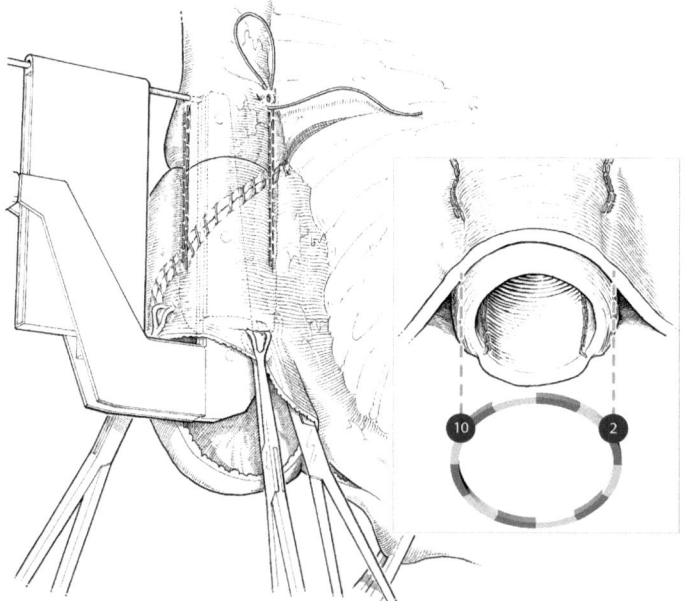

Fig. 6.8 Staple fixation of the anterior nipple valve to the anterior wall of the pouch at 10 and 2 o'clock using a TLH stapler. The puncture holes in the efferent limb from the pin of the stapler are closed with a purse string suture

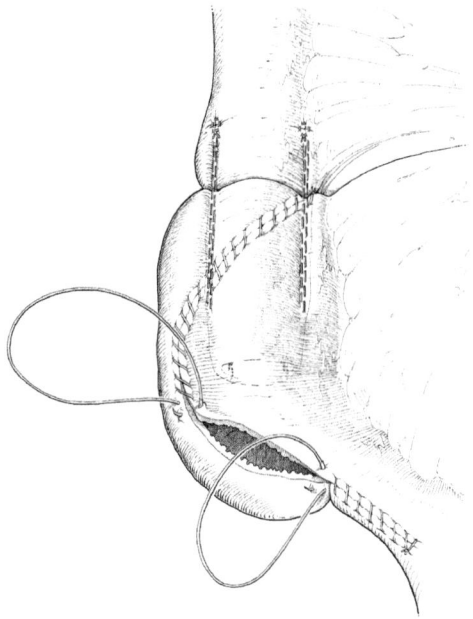

Fig. 6.9 Closure of the remaining anterior wall of the pouch in running fashion

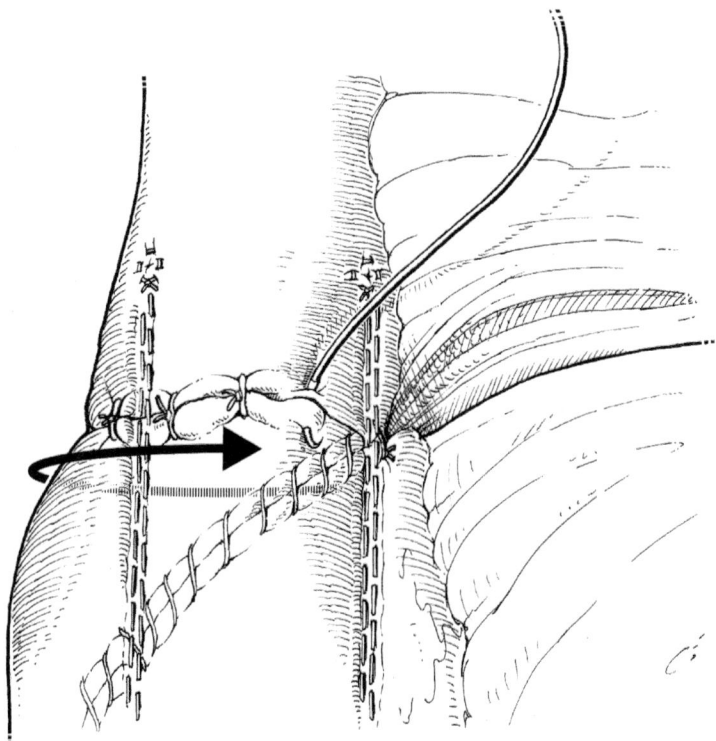

Fig. 6.10 Pouch cuff is secured to the efferent limb using circumferential interrupted sutures

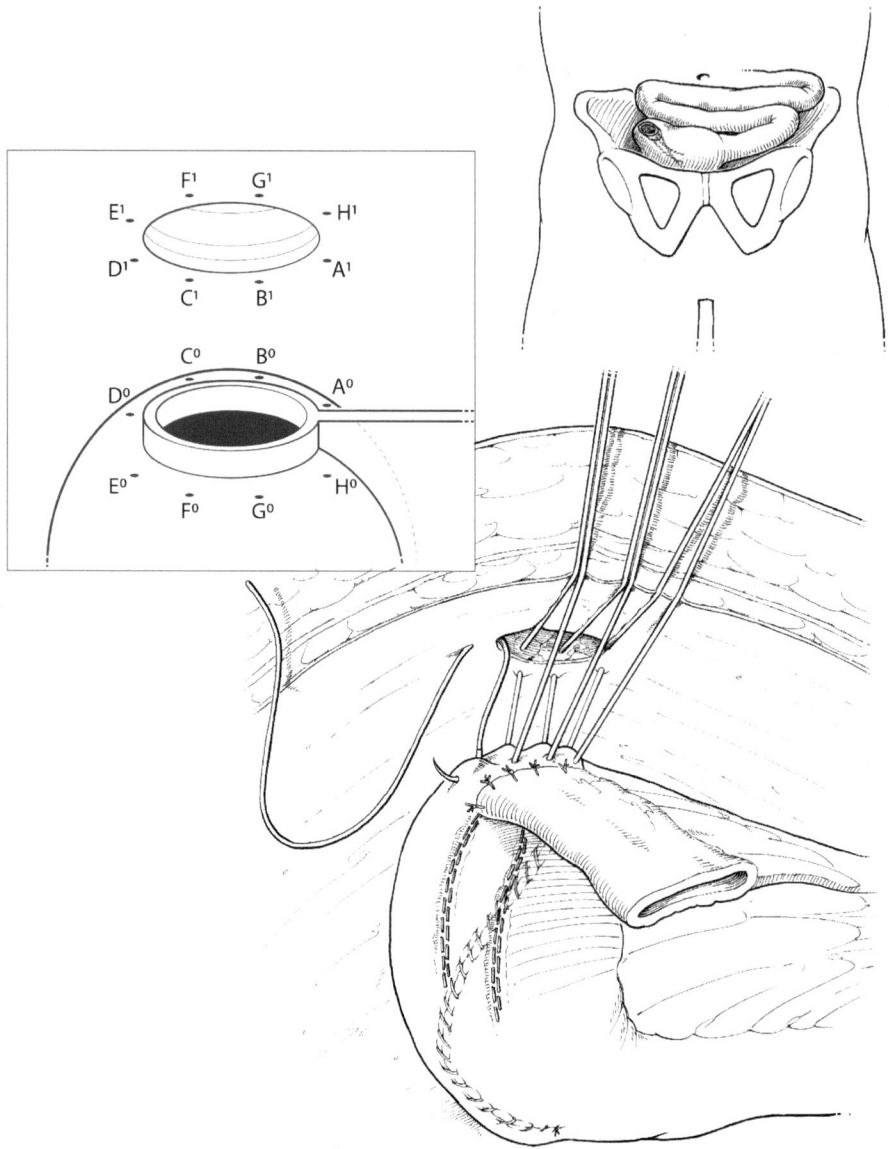

Fig. 6.11 The pouch is secured to the anterior abdominal wall at the level of the stomal orifice using interrupted sutures (see inset pouch placement in the lower abdomen and suture placement)

is supported by, the pelvic brim (inset, Fig. 6.11). A circular incision is then made for the stoma typically measuring only 2–3 cm in diameter. The pouch is then secured on the medial and lateral sides to the undersurface of the abdominal wall stomal opening, in order to mitigate the physical weight of the pouch pulling away from the wall posteriorly and inferiorly resulting in valve dessusception or slippage (Fig. 6.11). At this time, the pouch is tested again to ensure the Medina® catheter may easily cannulate the efferent limb and nipple, and to ensure continence once again. The redundant efferent limb is amputated at the level of, or just above the skin and secured (without eversion) to the skin with interrupted absorbable sutures.

Prior to re-inserting the Medina® catheter, a small segment of silicon tubing is placed over the medina catheter. The Medina® catheter is then reinserted into the pouch, confirming the position of the end of the tube within the pouch by palpation (rather than in the valve itself). Two sutures are then used to secure the tube in this position to the skin, and puncturing the silicon tubing rather than the Medina® catheter. The catheter is secured to a straight drainage bag. The midline incision is then closed in the usual fashion.

Post-operative management of the medina catheter is of utmost importance. For newly created pouches, the Medina® catheter is kept unclamped for 2 weeks to allow continuous drainage of the pouch. The catheter is irrigated with 50 ml of normal saline twice daily to keep it patent. The catheter itself has an opening at the bottom and two side holes. One should always check to ensure that the irrigation goes directly into the pouch itself. If fluid drains around the catheter, this indicates that the bottom hole of the catheter may be blocked, thus resulting in a complete bowel obstruction. Should this occur, the tube needs to be removed, cleaned, and reinserted. From postoperative weeks 2–4, clamping of the tube commences starting with clamping for 1 h out of every four gradually up to 3 h out of four; this allows the pouch to increase its capacity to accommodate effluent. At 4 weeks, the patient meets with our stoma nurse and is educated on how to intubate and irrigate the pouch and how to maintain the Medina® catheter.

6.3   Summary

Over the last 40 years, our approach to Kock pouch creation has evolved and adapted in an attempt to improve pouch function and reduce the need for revisional surgery. We believe that our current approach to Kock pouch creation provides a majority of patients with an excellent quality of life.

Bibliography

1. Kock NG. A new look at ileostomy. Surg Annu. 1976;8:241–56.
2. Go P. The continent ileostomy. Aalsmeer: Maastricht University; 1986.
3. Kock NG. Continent ileostomy. Prog Surg. 1973;12:180–201.
4. Bloemendaal AL, Lovegrove R, Buchs NC, Guy RJ, George BD. Continent ileostomy (Kock pouch) formation - a video vignette. Color Dis. 2017;19:85–6.
5. Fazio VW. Surgical management fo ulcerative colitis. In: Corman ML, editor. Corman's Colon and Rectal surgery. 6th ed. Philadelphia: Lippincott Williams & Wilkins; 2013.
6. Cohen Z. Current status of the continent ileostomy. Can J Surg. 1987;30(5):357–8.
7. Cohen Z. Evolution of the Kock continent reservoir ileostomy. Can J Surg. 1982;25(5):509–14.
8. Cohen Z, Stone RM. Continent reservoir ileostomy: 1. Early experience and evolution of the surgical technique. Can J Surg. 1980;23(3):259–62.

Chapter 7
Converting a Pelvic Pouch to a Kock Pouch

Jonas Bengtson and Anna Solberg

The majority of patients with a pelvic pouch have a good to excellent pouch function and health related quality of life. However, over 20% of the patients experience a poor functional outcome or a definite failure. Some complications could be managed with re-do pouch surgery, trans-anally with or without laparotomy. An alternative option to indefinite diversion or pouch excision is to convert the pelvic pouch to a continent ileostomy.

The main indication is the same as for the de novo construction; a patient with or without previous experience of stomal problems who will not accept a conventional end-ileostomy.

A very special indication for a conversion is when the pelvic pouch would not reach down to the ileoanal anastomosis. If this scenario has been discussed with the patient, it is possible to instead use the pelvic pouch to construct a continent ileostomy.

Information to the potential candidate for conversion should also include the important issue and the risk of loss of bowel length. It is reasonably well shown that even the loss of approximately 50 cm of small bowel could lead to clinically important metabolic disturbances including losses of electrolytes and water. The absolute ambition should therefore be to use the original (pelvic) pouch. Even if the outcome of conversion seems to be satisfying, there is inevitably a group of patients that in the future will end up with a definite failure also of the converted pouch. If this patient already had the pelvic pouch excised, the loss of 80 cm or more of small bowel is definitely a risk for some grade of intestinal failure.

There are a few publications, mainly small series, on conversion of the pelvic pouch to a continent pouch. Regarding the functional outcome, it appears to be satisfying, however with the price of a need of revisional surgery for many of the patients.

J. Bengtson (✉) · A. Solberg
Sahlgrenska University Hospital/Östra, Gothenburg, Sweden
e-mail: jonas.l.bengtsson@vgregion.se; anna.solberg@vgregion.se

© Springer Nature Switzerland AG 2019　　　　　　　　　　　　　　　　67
P. Myrelid, M. Block (eds.), *The Kock Pouch*,
https://doi.org/10.1007/978-3-319-95591-9_7

The first report on conversion of a malfunctioning pelvic pouch to a continent ileostomy was published in 1990 by Kusunoki et al., even though Hultén in 1985 mentioned the option of converting a malfunctioning pelvic pouch, but with no actual case described.

In 1992 Hultén et al. published results from Gothenburg were four out of five patients were continent. However, the follow-up time was not specified. The remaining patient had a nipple slipping and the pouch was subsequently converted to a conventional end-ileostomy.

The same patients were included in a later study published in 2004 from the Gothenburg group, now including 13 patients. Septic complications were the main reason for conversion in eight patients and poor function (mainly incontinence) for the remaining five. In all but one patient the original pelvic pouch was used for the reconstruction (Kock pouch). With a follow-up of median 6 years, 9 of the 10 patients with a functioning pouch was fully satisfied. Two patients had their pouch excised. One because of enterocutaneous fistula where the pathology report confirmed Crohn's disease and the other one with a motility disorder had the pouch excised after two unsuccessful revisisons. One patient was lost to follow-up.

Ecker et al. reported in 1996, conversion in five patients, all with functional problems. One patient with slow transit constipation as indication for proctocolectomy, had her Kock pouch excised because of abdominal pain of the same nature as she had with the pelvic pouch, relived only with permanent drainage of the pouch. Ecker also describes two types of modifications of the surgical procedure which will be briefly described below.

In the late 1990's Behrens et al. presented 42 patients from five centres in the US with pelvic pouch failure. The original pouch was used in only four of the patients, outcome data was not presented separately. Furthermore, all the patients were operated with the Barnet procedure.

In 2004 Karoui et al. presented the faith of seven patients who had their failed pelvic pouch converted to a Kock pouch. Five of these patients had their Kock pouch excised and the remaining two were waiting for pouch excision as well. One of the patients developed intestinal failure and was dependent on parenteral nutritional support.

The Cleveland Clinic, Ohio, US presented the so far largest series of 64 pouch conversions in 2009. The majority of the patients had septic complications as the main indication for conversion. However, in only 25% of the patients, the original pouch was used. These patients are not described in further detail, but did not differ regarding outcome. With a median follow-up of 5 years, 29 patients (45%) had Kock pouch revisions (the total number of procedures not reported). Slippage of the valve was the most common reason for surgery, with the same frequency whether original pouch were used or not. The pouch was excised in three patients due to septic and/or functional problems.

In Norway Wasmuth et al. presented the results from eleven conversions were the cause of pelvic pouch failure was due to septic complications in six patients and incontinence in three. The pelvic pouch was used in seven patients. With a median follow-up of 7 years, two patients had their Kock pouch excised due to fistula and on one of them slipping of the nipple valve as well. Of the remaining nine patients, all were satisfied, eight fully continent and one patient suffered minor leakage. One of these patients needed further revisional Kock pouch surgery due to valve slippage combined with detachment from the abdominal wall. The authors concluded that the surgical burden on patients with a Kock pouch formation after failed pelvic pouch is no higher than expected for Kock pouch surgery in general and the success rate is high.

7.1   Patient Selection

Patients with septic complications involving the ileo-anal anastomosis that is not suitable for, or were salvage surgery has failed, could be candidates for conversion a Kock pouch. Another group of patients are those with functional problems as for example incontinence, urgency or increased frequency of bowel movements.

Contraindications, absolute or relative, to a conversion are in principle the same as for the de-novo Kock pouch. Mental disability, grave obesity, serious comorbidity, Crohn's disease of the small bowel, and a manifest or impending intestinal failure are not suitable. Likewise, chronic pouchitis are probably at least a relative contraindication to a conversion.

7.2   The Conversion Procedure

For patients with septic complications, everything possible should be done to make the conditions as aseptic as possible. This implies of course optimal drainage of abscesses and/or fistulas and in some cases, to achieve this, also a diverting stoma.

The primary goal for the first part of the operation should be to do the dissection as atraumatic as possible in order to save the original pelvic pouch and to minimize damage to the pelvic nerves. The most troublesome part is obviously in the deep pelvis, especially in the male pelvis. Beside the visibility, potential sepsis in proximity to the pelvic pouch tends to make the right dissection planes hard or even impossible to define. Sometimes a simultaneous dissection from below could be of great help. Furthermore, minor damage to the pouch is not a disaster, as it most often tends to happen in the area of the ileo-anal anastomosis. Accordingly, it could be incorporated in the creation of the new inlet. However, major injuries to the body of the pelvic pouch itself necessitates the construction of a de novo Kock pouch.

The defect at the former ileo-anal anastomosis is taken care of in a conventional manner. It is most often enough to do an intersphincteric resection and not necessary a formal amputation. If there is fistula, it is often wise to let parts of the wound lay open for secondary healing to minimize the risk of postoperative septic complications.

The continent ileostomy is principally constructed in the same way as for a rotation of the pouch described in Chap. 17.

It is often convenient to use the former outlet for the anastomosis of the new inlet. In the case of a severely damaged outlet, it could be a better option to close this area and make an incision in a more remote area for the new inlet. The pouch is placed and anchored to the abdominal wall as for a de novo Kock pouch.

Standard conversion of a pelvic pouch to a continent ileostomy

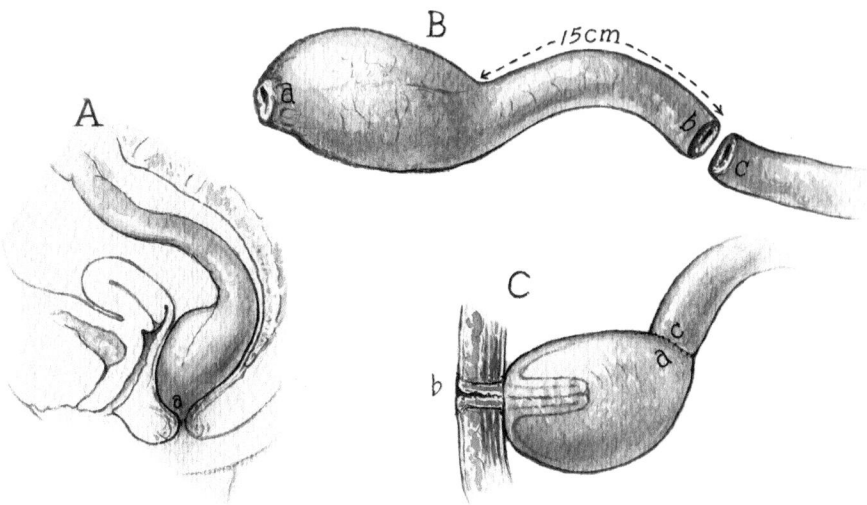

Ecker described an alternative construction for two special situations. If the capacity of the pouch was insufficient, the oral ileum was anastomosed side-to-side with the two-loop J-pouch, this augmentation forming almost a three-loop S-pouch.

If the pouch capacity was too large, the afferent loop was also dilated and could not be used to form the valve. In this case, the valve was formed from a higher, normal caliber ileal segment and transposed into the former pouch outlet, and intestinal continuity was re-established by entero-anastomosis between oral ileum and the afferent loop.

Especially the second situation has in our experience been viewed as a potential problem. We have in these cases made a conventional rotation of the Kock pouch with the argument that the bowel dilatation probably will diminish when the relative obstruction is relieved. For a few of these patients, subsequent slipping of the nipple valve has occurred, but without obvious signs of a markedly floppy nipple endoscopically or at revisional surgery. However, there has been a suspicion that the dilated nipple segment may have contributed to the complication.

7.3   Conclusion

Conversion of the pelvic pouch is definitely an option for a group of patients with pelvic pouch failure. Counseling the patient in this scenario is of course crucial, as there is a major risk of additional procedures and in the long run a definite failure. In our view, the goal should be to save the primary pouch, which technically tends to be one of the most difficult parts of the procedure. For a colorectal surgical team highly experienced with Kock pouch surgery as well as with re-do pelvic pouch surgery it is however achievable.

Bibliography

1. Behrens DT, et al. Conversion of failed ileal pouch-anal anastomosis to continent ileostomy. Dis Colon Rectum. 1999;42(4):490–5. discussion 495-496.
2. Borjesson L, et al. The failed pelvic pouch: conversion to a continent ileostomy. Tech Coloproctol. 2004;8(2):102–5.
3. Delin K, et al. Factors regulating sodium balance in proctocolectomized patients with various ileal resections. Scand J Gastroenterol. 1984;19(2):145–9.
4. Kusunoki M, et al. Conversion of malfunctioning J pouch to Kock's pouch. Case report. Acta Chir Scand. 1990;156(2):179–81.
5. Ecker KW, et al. Conversion of the failing ileoanal pouch to reservoir-ileostomy rather than to ileostomy alone. Dis Colon Rectum. 1996;39(9):977–80.
6. Hulten L, et al. The failing pelvic pouch conversion to continent ileostomy. Int J Color Dis. 1992;7(3):119–21.
7. Karoui M, et al. Results of surgical removal of the pouch after failed restorative proctocolectomy. Dis Colon Rectum. 2004;47(6):869–75.
8. Lian L, et al. Outcomes for patients undergoing continent ileostomy after a failed ileal pouch-anal anastomosis. Dis Colon Rectum. 2009;52(8):1409–14. discussion 4414-1406.
9. Parc Y, et al. The continent ileostomy: an alternative to end ileostomy? Short and long-term results of a single institution series. Dig Liver Dis. 2011;43(10):779–83.
10. Wasmuth HH, et al. Failed pelvic pouch substituted by continent ileostomy. Color Dis. 2010;12(7 Online):e109–13.

Chapter 8
Kock Pouch as a Pelvic Pouch

Mattias Block

8.1 Introduction

There have been different methods and techniques described throughout history in creating the pelvic pouch or ileal pouch-anal anastomosis, starting with the *S*-pouch (Fig. 8.1) by Sir Alan Parks and John Nicolls at St Marks Hospital in London in the late 1970s. Functional outcome was reported as good, except for problems with pouch emptying; more than 50% of the patients had to use a catheter for evacuation. This was due to the long pouch outlet in the initial design, the so-called *S*-pouch (Fig. 8.1).

Shortly thereafter John Nicholls constructed the *W*-pouch (Fig. 8.2) which demanded much more bowel length and more suture lines. Utsunomiya from Japan soon thereafter (in the early 1980's) constructed the *J*-pouch (Fig. 8.3a, b) which is a simple and straight-forward technique, nowadays by far the most used technique world-wide. An alternative method to construct the pelvic pouch originated from Gothenburg, Sweden and was created from the same technique as when creating the continent ileostomy (Kock pouch) but omitting the nipple valve (Fig. 8.3a, c).

The theoretical advantage of a *K*-pouch is that it develops into a spherical rather than a cylindrical design, resulting in a proportionally larger volume for the length of ileum used. Furthermore, the *K*-pouch reduces the dead space in the small pelvis and there is some evidence that the *K*-pouch (as well as the *W*-pouch) could have a slightly superior function. Usually, the pelvic pouch is performed with a diverting temporary loop ileostomy as part of the procedure, but in selected cases it may be omitted.

M. Block (✉)
Department of Surgery, Sahlgrenska University Hospital, University of Gothenburg, Gothenburg, Sweden
e-mail: mattias.block@vgregion.se

© Springer Nature Switzerland AG 2019
P. Myrelid, M. Block (eds.), *The Kock Pouch*,
https://doi.org/10.1007/978-3-319-95591-9_8

Fig. 8.1 *S*-pouch

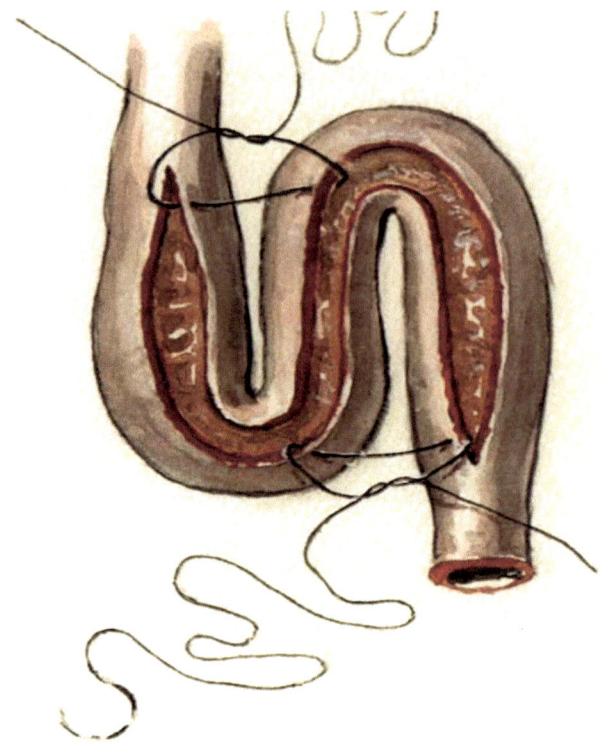

Fig. 8.2 *W*-pouch

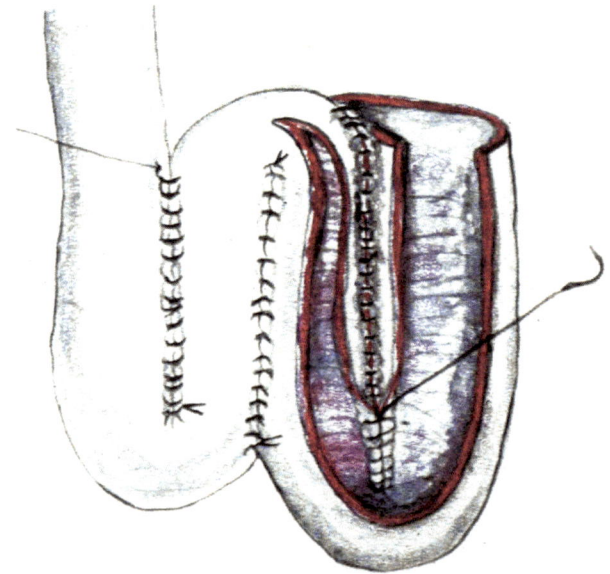

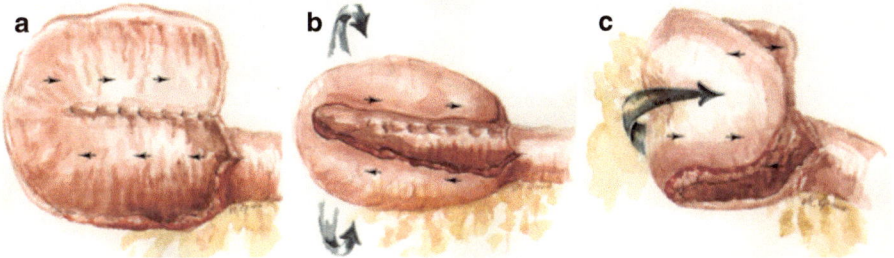

Fig. 8.3 Construction of the pelvic pouch. (**a**) First step. (**b**) *J*-pouch. (**c**) *K*-pouch

When comparing the *J*-pouch to the *K*-pouch, the *J*-pouch consist of 2 × 15 cm of the terminal ileum stapled together at the anti-mesenteric side, creating a banana-like shape and the anvil of the circular stapler is placed in the apex of the reservoir (Fig. 8.3a, b).

The *K*-pouch also consist of 2 × 15 cm of the ileum. The construction start exactly as when constructing the continent ileostomy, however, the 15 cm of the distal end used to construct the nipple valve in the continent ileostomy is left out (Fig. 8.3a, c). After putting the 2 × 15 cm of distal ileum next to each-other, the bowel is opened op and the back wall is suture with continuous absorbable mono-filament 4.0 suture (Fig. 8.4a–c). At the apex of the reservoir interrupted sutures are put of approximately 3–4 cm length. This is where the anvil of circular stapler later is inserted into the reservoir. The two sides of the front wall of the bowel are then folded up toward the afferent limb and sutured with the same technique as used at the back wall. This way a more pear-like shape compared to the J-pouch is constructed.

After finishing the suturing of the pouch it is pushed through the mesentery (a maneuver that has to be seen live to be fully understood) and the construction of the reservoir is then completed (Fig. 8.4d–g).

The *K*-reservoir creates a larger volume than the *J*-reservoir, especially initially at time of the construction of the pouch. Studies have shown that the volume after some time gets more similar but still a slight difference remains, in favor of the *K*-reservoir. Theoretically, this could bring better capacity to the *K*-reservoir and so forth better functional outcome, which has been shown by some authors. At least, the *K*-reservoir is not inferior in functional outcome compared to the *J*-reservoir.

In addition, being a centre performing continent ileostomies (Kock pouch) creating the *K*-reservoir gives surgeons good training in performing Kock pouches since the technique is very similar, as described above.

One disadvantage of the technique is that it takes longer time to construct (an additional 45 min operating time) compared to the *J*-reservoir. It is technically more demanding with more steps, and not as easy to reproduce, as the *J*-reservoir. However, the pelvic *K*-reservoir has its place in advanced restorative proctocolectomy.

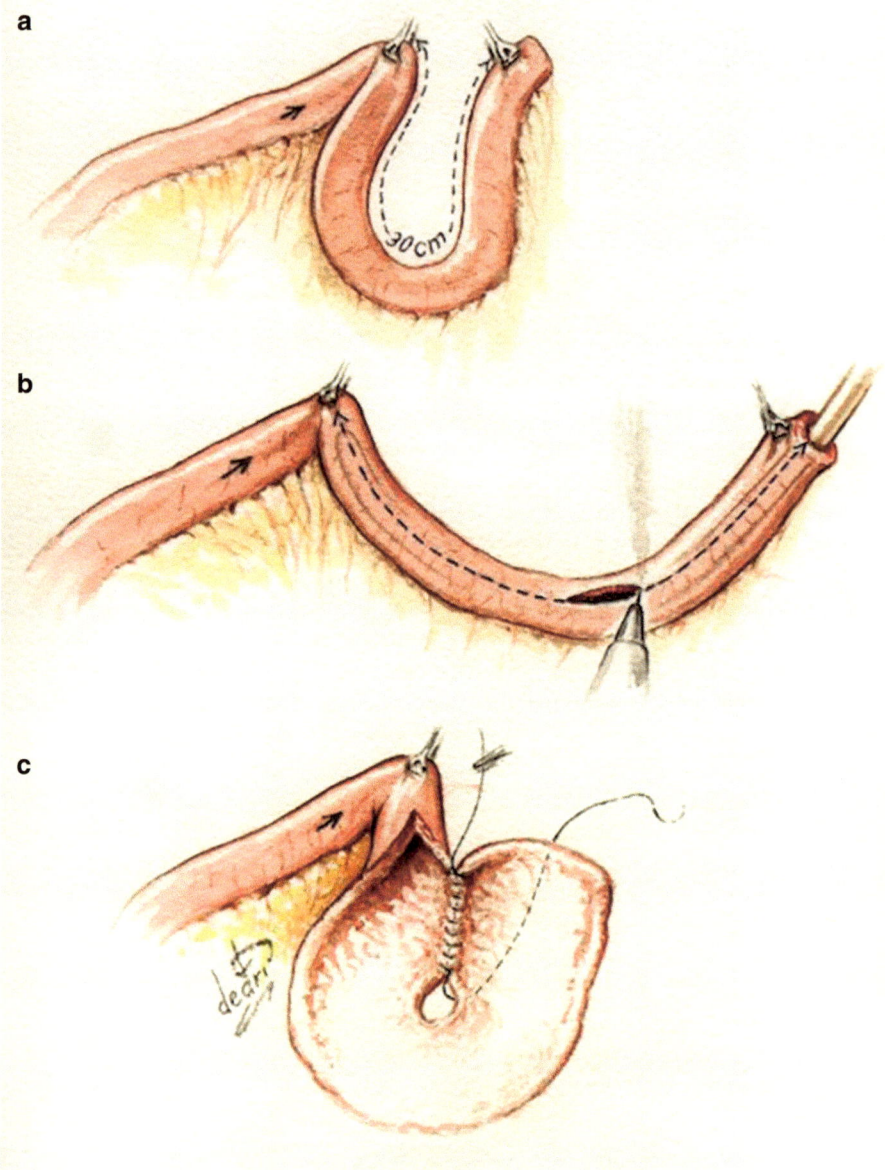

Fig. 8.4 (**a–c**) Construction of a pelvic K-pouch, part one. (**a**) Distal 30 cm of ileum is laid side-by-side (2 × 15 cm). (**b**) The bowel is opened with cautery. (**c**) The back wall is sutured with continuous 4.0 sutures. The last 3–4 cm are sutured with interrupted sutures due to placement of the anvil at the apex of the reservoir. (**d–g**) Construction of a pelvic K-pouch, part two. (**d**) The front wall of the bowel is folded up towards the afferent limb and sutured with two separate lines of continuous 4.0 sutures. (**e–f**) The corners of the pouch are now pushed through the mesentery (a maneuver that has to be seen live to be fully understood). (**g**) The pouch is constructed with a pear-like shape. A hand-sewn pouch anal anastomosis is shown and the suture marks the place of this anastomosis. In a sta-pled anastomosis the anvil comes out at the apex of the, e.g. the location of the suture

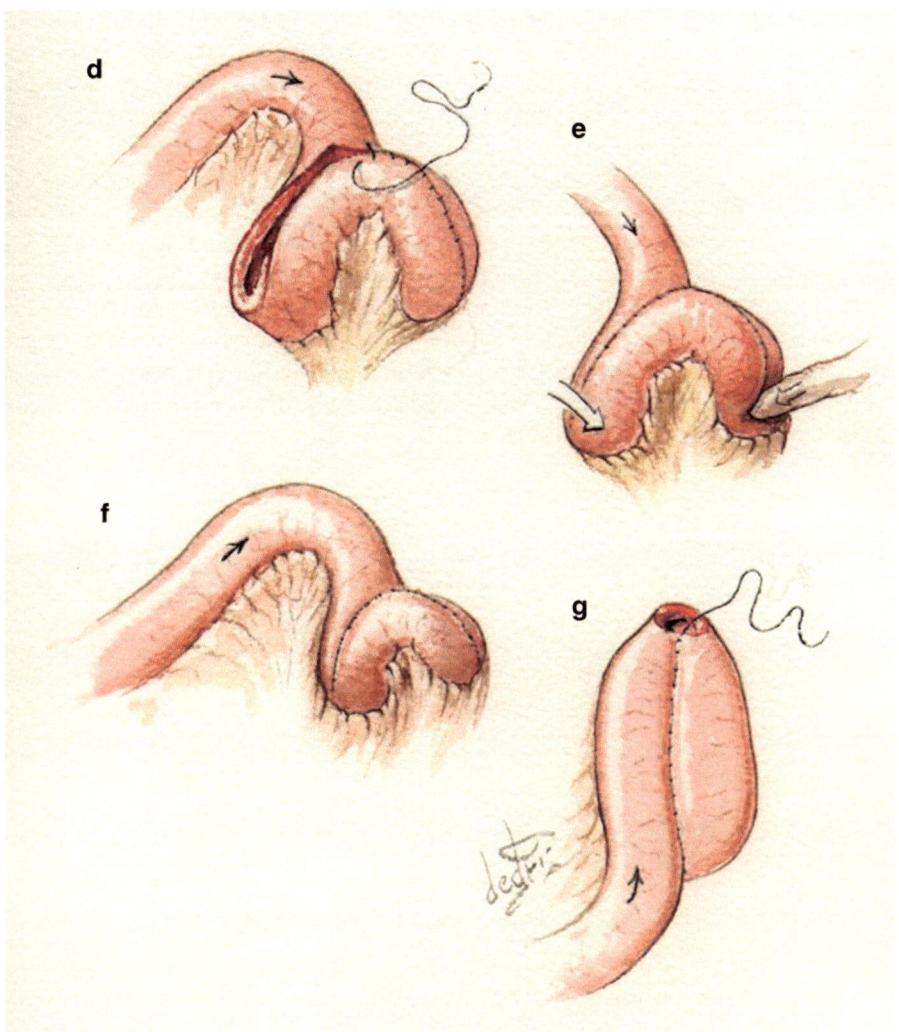

Fig. 8.4 (continued)

The **K**-pouch may be described as a double-folded **J**-pouch, according to the technique used for constructing a continent ileostomy. It is reasonable to assume that the **K**-pouch shares many of the features of the **W**-pouch, which may also be described as a double-folded **J**-pouch. We have previously described the functional outcome and manovolumetric characteristics of the **K**-pouch in comparison to the **J**-pouch. The **K**-pouch was found to achieve around 30% more volume than the **J**-pouch. One explanation for this fact is that, when distended, the **K**-pouch adopts a more sphere-like shape, while the **J**-pouch becomes cylinder-shaped, which has an inherently smaller volume.

Some authors have shown that the *K*-pouch is associated with slightly superior long term function, principally regarding continence. This is somewhat surprising, since previous data suggests that the superiority of the *K*-pouch is related to its larger volume and hence logically to stool frequency rather than continence. A possible explanation for this may be that the *K*-pouch exerts less strain on the continence mechanisms.

It would be a bold statement to recommend all colleagues of the international colorectal surgical community to perform *K*-pouches as standard procedure in pelvic pouches. Compared to the *J*-pouch, the *K*-pouch is technically more complex to perform. Introduction of the procedure could be associated with complications during the learning curve. However, in a unit that regularly performs continent ileostomies it is an excellent way to keep up the competence for this procedure, since pelvic pouch with a *K*-design is constructed in the same manner as a continent ileostomy (omitting the nipple segment).

Bibliography

1. Parks AG, Nicholls RJ. Proctocolectomy without ileostomy for ulcerative colitis. Br Med J. 1978;2(6130):85–8.
2. Utsunomiya J, Iwama T, Imajo M, et al. Total colectomy, mucosal proctectomy, and ileoanal anastomosis. Dis Colon Rectum. 1980;23(7):459–66.
3. Kock NG. Intra-abdominal "reservoir" in patients with permanent ileostomy. Preliminary observations on a procedure resulting in fecal "continence" in five ileostomy patients. Arch Surg. 1969;99(2):223–31.
4. Sunde ML, Øresland T, Faerden AE. Restorative proctocolectomy with two different pouch designs: few complications with good function. Color Dis. 2017;19(4):363–71. https://doi.org/10.1111/codi.13478.
5. Lovegrove RE, Heriot AG, Constantinides V, et al. Meta-analysis of short-term and long-term outcomes of J, W and S ileal reservoirs for restorative proctocolectomy. Color Dis. 2007;9(4):310–20.
6. Ravitch MM, Sabiston DC Jr. Anal ileostomy with preservation of the sphincter; a proposed operation in patients requiring total colectomy for benign lesions. Surg Gynecol Obstet. 1947;84(6):1095–9.
7. Drobni S. One-stage proctocolectomy and anal ileostomy: report of 35 cases. Dis Colon Rectum. 1967;10(6):443–8.
8. Goligher JC. The functional results after sphincter-saving resections of the rectum. Ann R Coll Surg Engl. 1951;8(6):421–38.
9. Valiente MA, Bacon HE. Construction of pouch using pantaloon technic for pull-through of ileum following total colectomy; report of experimental work and results. Am J Surg. 1955;90(5):742–50.
10. Nicholls RJ, Pezim ME. Restorative proctocolectomy with ileal reservoir for ulcerative colitis and familial adenomatous polyposis: a comparison of three reservoir designs. Br J Surg. 1985a;72(6):470–4.
11. Kock NG, Hulten L, Myrvold HE. Ileoanal anastomosis with interposition of the ileal 'Kock pouch'. Preliminary results. Dis Colon Rectum. 1989;32(12):1050–4.
12. Joyce MR, Kiran RP, Remzi FH, Church J, Fazio VW. In a select group of patients meeting strict clinical criteria and undergoing ileal pouch-anal anastomosis, the omission of a diverting ileostomy offers cost savings to the hospital. Dis Colon Rectum. 2010;53(6):905–10.

13. Remzi FH, Fazio VW, Gorgun E, et al. The outcome after restorative proctocolectomy with or without defunctioning ileostomy. Dis Colon Rectum. 2006;49(4):470–7.
14. Bach SP, Mortensen NJ. Revolution and evolution: 30 years of ileoanal pouch surgery. Inflamm Bowel Dis. 2006;12(2):131–45.
15. Heald RJ, Allen DR. Stapled ileo-anal anastomosis: a technique to avoid mucosal proctectomy in the ileal pouch operation. Br J Surg. 1986;73(7):571–2.
16. Borjesson L, Oresland T, Hulten L. The failed pelvic pouch: conversion to a continent ileostomy. Tech Coloproctol. 2004;8(2):102–5.
17. Chapman JR, Larson DW, Wolff BG, et al. Ileal pouch-anal anastomosis: does age at the time of surgery affect outcome? Arch Surg. 2005;140(6):534–9. discussion 9-40.
18. Michelassi F, Lee J, Rubin M, et al. Long-term functional results after ileal pouch anal restorative proctocolectomy for ulcerative colitis: a prospective observational study. Ann Surg. 2003;238(3):433–41. discussion 42-5.
19. Erkek AB, Remzi FH, Hammel JP, Akyuz M, Fazio VW. Effect of small bowel obstruction on functional outcome and quality of life in patients with ileal pouch-anal anastomosis: 10-year follow-up study. J Gastroenterol Hepatol. 2008;23(1):119–25.
20. Hallberg H, Stahlberg D, Akerlund JE. Ileal pouch-anal anastomosis (IPAA): functional outcome after postoperative pelvic sepsis. A prospective study of 100 patients. Int J Color Dis. 2005;20(6):529–33.
21. Mikkola K, Luukkonen P, Jarvinen HJ. Long-term results of restorative proctocolectomy for ulcerative colitis. Int J Color Dis. 1995;10(1):10–4.
22. Ogunbiyi OA, Korsgen S, Keighley MR. Pouch salvage. Long-term outcome. Dis Colon Rectum. 1997;40(5):548–52.
23. Akbari RP, Madoff RD, Parker SC, et al. Anastomotic sinuses after ileoanal pouch construction: incidence, management, and outcome. Dis Colon Rectum. 2009;52(3):452–5.
24. Sagar PM, Lewis W, Holdsworth PJ, Johnston D. One-stage restorative proctocolectomy without temporary defunctioning ileostomy. Dis Colon Rectum. 1992;35(6):582–8.
25. Nicholls RJ, Pezim ME. Restorative proctocolectomy with ileal reservoir for ulcerative colitis and familial adenomatous polyposis: a comparison of 3 reservoir designs. Br J Surg. 1985b;72:470–4.

Chapter 9
Post-operative Care

Pär Myrelid

Just like in any colorectal surgical procedure you need to have a patient fit for surgery with optimized physiological conditions. The creation of the Kock pouch itself includes a lot of suture lines that have to heal properly and thus the risks of a leak are too high in a patient not physiologically suited for this kind of surgery. This is especially true if there will be a blockage of the draining catheter as the created nipple valve of the pouch causes a small bowel obstruction, with even higher pressure on the suture lines of the pouch.

Patients are given peri-operative anti-thrombosis prophylaxis in line with standard colorectal procedures as well as antibiotic prophylaxis. Sometimes the antibiotic prophylaxis is extended for about 1–3 days, depending on the level of spillage of bowel content per-operatively. Pain relief is preferable given through an epidural catheter for a few days and then changed to standard post-operative pain relief. Apart from the care of the pouch itself the use of a standard enhanced recovery program for colorectal surgery may be used letting the patient eat and drink ad libitum, as long as there are no signs of complications.

The main concern in the peri-operative phase is the Kock pouch itself. The two main concerns are an anastomotic leak from the long suture lines and blockage of the draining catheter, which in itself can cause a leak from the suture lines. In theatre the surgeon has to make sure the draining catheter is properly positioned. The catheter should be positioned with the tip beyond the nipple valve but without pushing toward the bowel wall at the bottom of the pouch. When positioned it should be secured with sutures from the peri-stomal skin and tied around the catheter and then further secured with bandage (see Chap. 11).

The Kock pouch catheter should be left in place and continuously draining for the first 2 weeks. During the first 24 h the Kock pouch should be flushed with

P. Myrelid (✉)
Linköping University Hospital, Department of Surgery, Linköping University, Department of Clinical and Experimental Medicine, Linköping, Sweden
e-mail: par.myrelid@liu.se

© Springer Nature Switzerland AG 2019
P. Myrelid, M. Block (eds.), *The Kock Pouch*,
https://doi.org/10.1007/978-3-319-95591-9_9

50–100 ml saline every fourth hour and thereafter every sixth hour for the rest of the 2 weeks, but by then lukewarm water could be used instead of saline. During the third and fourth post-operative week the catheter could be spigoted and flushed regularly during daytime while left open and continuously draining night-time. Flushing should be done slowly and the output of fluid afterwards should be bile colored, as a sign of the catheter properly draining the pouch. Do not use suction by a syringe, rather let the pouch drain passively. If the post-operative course is uneventful the patient can usually leave the hospital after about 1–2 weeks.

Everyone involved in the care of the patient must be aware of these risks and follow a strict post-operative regimen. One way of making sure of this is to have clear instructions following the patient at all time after the surgery. A step by step list for troubleshooting may be a useful tool (Table 9.1). This list should involve a brief explanation of the procedure and a manual of the care of the

Table 9.1 A step by step troubleshooting list in the post-operative period in the event of a discontinued drainage from the Kock pouch

1. The Kock pouch is drained by a catheter during the healing phase of 4–5 weeks. The catheter should during that time be completely open and draining continuously to a bag for 2 weeks. During the third and fourth week the catheter can be spigoted during day time and rinsed at least every fourth hour. During night time the catheter should be left open and continuously draining again to the bag.

2. The most important role for the catheter is to make sure the pouch is not expanded too much by the luminal content. Thus it is of the utmost importance that the catheter is draining properly.

3. The Kock pouch should be flushed by 50–100 ml of saline every fourth hour the first 24 h. Thereafter the flushing could be extended to every sixth hour for the following 2 weeks.

4. When flushing do it slowly and make sure the output afterwards is bile colored, as a sign of the catheter properly draining the pouch. Do not use suction by the syringe, rather let it drain passively.

5. In case of uncertainty flush with another 50 ml of saline. One cause of malfunctioning could be that the position of the catheter has been altered, e.g. the catheter is inside of the nipple rather than going through the nipple into the pouch. Another reason may be that the openings of the draining catheter are blocked by luminal content or by the mucosa of the pouch wall. Reposition of the catheter 1–2 cm, or as much as the anchoring stiches will let you, and see if that will help the draining.

6. If the taken measures above have not solved the problem with the non-draining catheter call the responsible surgeon or the on call surgeon to do the actions below.

7. Sweep the draining catheter by putting a thinner catheter inside, e.g. a LoFric® catheter or similar (Fig. 9.1). The thinner catheter must be long enough to go through the tip of the bent Kock pouch catheter. If you are not sure it is long enough compare with another bent Kock pouch catheter (usually 30 cm long).

8. If the sweeping action does not help you need to change the Kock pouch catheter itself. Cut the anchoring stiches. Put a soft tip guide wire through the Kock pouch catheter and make sure it is well inside the pouch and then remove the Kock pouch catheter. Use lots of lubricants when putting the new Kock pouch catheter over the guide wire and into the pouch. Remember that the catheter must pass through the whole abdominal wall (usually about at least 3 cm) and thereafter the nipple valve (usually about an additional 5 cm) before the tip has entered the pouch and the draining is resumed.

Fig. 9.1 A LoFric® catheter can be used for sweeping a blocked Kock catheter. Make sure it is thin enough to go through the Kock catheter and long enough to pass the tip of the Kock catheter

Fig. 9.2 A Straight Kock catheter is used by the patient after the first 4 weeks has passed after the surgery. Before that a U-shaped (bent) Kock catheter is secured by anchoring stiches and/or tape to make sure the pouch is well drained

pouch in order to prevent as well as dealing with potential problems. It is important to make sure there is a spare U-shaped Kock pouch catheter as well as a thinner and longer catheter kept together with the patient in case of blockage of the drainage (Fig. 9.1).

The first step if it is uncertain, or obvious, that the catheter is not draining properly is to flush with another 50 ml of saline. Luminal content can cause blockage of the catheter and is usually solved with such extra flushing, by dilution of the luminal content. Other causes of malfunctioning could be that the position of the catheter has been altered, e.g. the catheter is inside of the nipple rather than going through the nipple into the pouch or the openings of the draining catheter are tilting against the pouch wall. Reposition of the catheter 1–2 cm, or as much as the anchoring stiches will allow, may restore the draining. If these measures does not re-establish the passive drainage the next step is by trying to sweep the Kock catheter by putting a thinner catheter inside of it, e.g. a LoFric® catheter or similar (Fig. 9.1). This thinner catheter must be long enough to go through the tip of the U-shaped Kock pouch catheter. This could be done by comparing with another U-shaped Kock pouch catheter (usually 30 cm long). If the sweeping action does not help it is necessary to change the Kock pouch catheter itself. This is done by cutting the anchoring stiches followed by introduction of a soft tip guide wire through the Kock pouch catheter. It should be made sure that the guide wire is well inside the pouch before removing the Kock pouch catheter itself. A fair amount of lubricants should be used when putting a new Kock pouch catheter over the guide wire and into the pouch. The catheter must pass through the whole abdominal wall (usually about at least 3 cm) and thereafter the nipple valve (usually about an additional 5 cm) before the tip has entered the pouch and the draining is resumed.

In case of an anastomotic leak the patient should be treated in the same manner as any patient with a leaking colorectal anastomosis. However, in many cases the leaking pouch can be rescued by over-sewing the leaking suture line and at the same time creating a diverting loop ileostomy as close as possible to the Kock pouch. In the case of severe leakages, ischemia of the pouch itself or necrosis of the nipple valve it may be necessary to remove the pouch (Fig. 9.3). In such a case one should refrain from further repair and rather give the patient an end ileostomy and, if possible, offer the patient another attempt at a later stage.

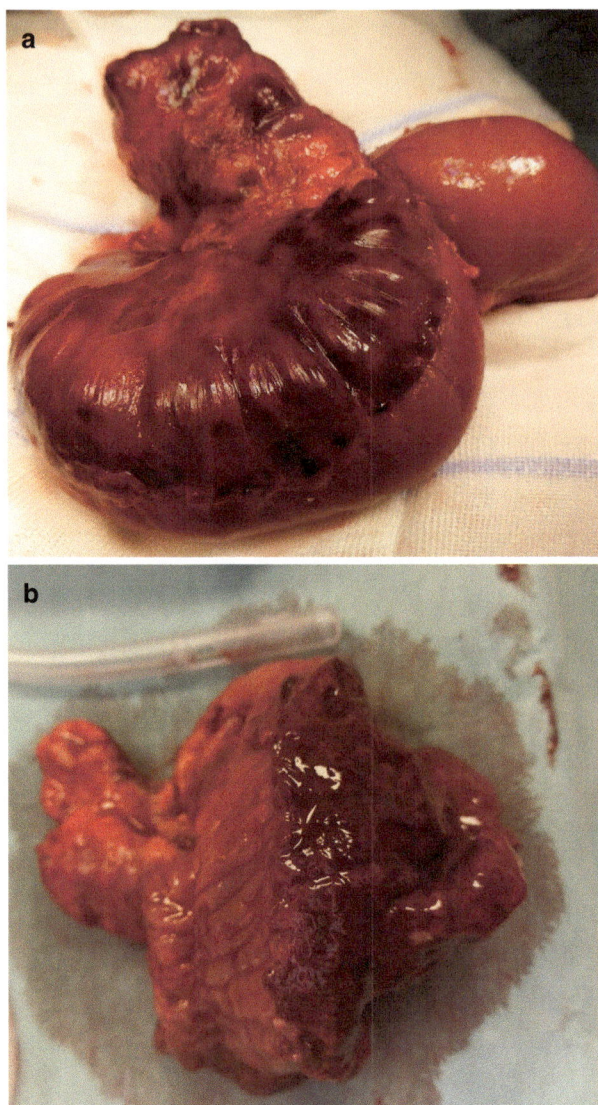

Fig. 9.3 A Kock pouch with venous stasis causing necrosis of half of the pouch necessitating exstirpation and creation of an end ileostomy. First picture of the exterior (**a**) and the second of the interior of the pouch (**b**)

9.1 Late Post-Operative Care

Approximately 4 weeks post-operatively the patient is taken back to the outpatient clinic and the catheter is removed. The patient catheterizes him−/her-self the first time together with the surgeon and/or stoma therapist. If the patient has travelled a long distance it usually feels good if the patient leaves the hospital for a few hours before coming back and making sure the emptying procedure works well. The next step is to make sure the pouch slowly increases in size and volume using a scheme with increasing length of time between each emptying (see Chap. 11).

Bibliography

1. Spinelli A, et al. Review article: optimal preparation for surgery in Crohn's disease. Aliment Pharmacol Ther. 2014;40(9):1009–22.
2. Gross ME, et al. The importance of extended postoperative venous thromboembolism prophylaxis in IBD: a National Surgical Quality Improvement Program analysis. Dis Colon Rectum. 2014;57(4):482–9.
3. Rawlinson A, et al. A systematic review of enhanced recovery protocols in colorectal surgery. Ann R Coll Surg Engl. 2011;93(8):583–8.
4. Kariv Y, et al. Clinical outcomes and cost analysis of a "fast track" postoperative care pathway for ileal pouch-anal anastomosis: a case control study. Dis Colon Rectum. 2007;50(2):137–46.
5. Dozois RR, et al. Improved results with continent ileostomy. Ann Surg. 1980;192(3):319–24.
6. Mergener K. Endoscopic management of Kock pouch dysfunction: case report of a method to establish wire-guided pouch access for catheterization. Gastrointest Endosc. 2003;57(6):780–2.

Chapter 10
Early Post Operative Complications

Neil Mortensen

Creation of a Kock pouch is a major intra-abdominal procedure and patients have often had major abdominal surgery previously. Complications are not uncommon and early complications will particularly be considered here. These can include those of any operation such as anaesthetic problems, chest or urinary tract infection as well as deep vein thrombosis.

Reoperative surgery can give rise to adhesional obstruction, and an inadvertent small bowel injury with an abscess or enteric fistula. There are particular problems related to the post-operative intubation of the pouch.

The specific early complications of a Kock pouch are related to the creation of the pouch and the valve.

10.1 Early Post-operative Pouch Catheter Problems

Patients are offered liquids when they are hungry and solid food when there is gas, or intestinal content starting to drain from their pouch catheter. The pouch is left on continuous gravity drainage for 2 weeks. Patients are then instructed on catheter management and taught how to insert their drainage catheter after 4 weeks. We use a Medina® catheter. After this period the patients gradually extend the time they leave the catheter out. So the catheter can inadvertently fall out during the 2 week 'quarantine' period and it is important to replace it as soon as possible. If the catheter cannot be simply replaced there may need to be assistance using a bougie, paediatric gastroscope with minimal insufflation and if need be a guide wire. Early blockage of the catheter can be managed with irrigation, or replacement.

N. Mortensen (✉)
Oxford University Hospitals, University of Oxford, Oxford, UK
e-mail: neil.mortensen@nds.ox.ac.uk

© Springer Nature Switzerland AG 2019
P. Myrelid, M. Block (eds.), *The Kock Pouch*,
https://doi.org/10.1007/978-3-319-95591-9_10

10.2   Bleeding

There are numerous suture lines and the knife-less staple lines of the valve, and these can all bleed. This will be obvious from the post operative indwelling catheter unless it becomes blocked. The classical signs of bleeding with a rising pulse and falling blood pressure should raise suspicion of an intra-pouch or intra- peritoneal bleed. With blood in the catheter an immediate pouchoscopy is indicated if an initial period of conservative management with intravenous fluids and blood transfusion is ineffective. The pouch should be washed out with saline via the pouch catheter and an endoscope passed in to the pouch. Some use a mixture of saline and adrenaline. If the bleeding site can be identified all the usual techniques for endoscopic therapy can be used including diathermy, clips, an injection of adrenaline or compression. If this fails or the bleeding is intraperitoneal consideration should be given to interventional radiography and selective angio occlusion with coils or sponge. As a last resort a further laparotomy may be necessary.

10.3   Suture Line Leakage and Peritonitis

It is in some ways surprising this does not happen more often given the long suture lines constructed by hand and at risk. The pouch is defunctioned and decompressed by the post op pouch catheter so minor leaks may be subclinical and not come to much. In patients with pain out of proportion to their general state, a change in vital signs or a rising C-reactive protein an immediate CT scan with intra-pouch and intravenous contrast is indicated. These patients already have a potentially compromised small bowel length so there is no excuse for delay. A small localised collection can be managed by percutaneous drainage but otherwise so much is at stake that an early laparotomy and intervention is mandatory within the first 10–12 days post op. The abdomen needs to be drained, lavaged and the leakage site repaired. An air water bubble leakage test may be useful. If there is any doubt about the repair or the site an upstream defunctioning ileostomy should be raised. This may avoid the development of an intestinal fistula.

10.4   Valve Necrosis

The use of the knifeless linear stapler has undoubtedly been a major step forward but using four throws or three with one misplaced along the mesentery can rarely result in a catastrophe, namely necrosis of the valve. Whilst it is not uncommon to see a rather black and blue nipple valve immediately after construction this is the extreme which does not pink up, become oedematous and then settle. The onset of symptoms can be slow and insidious, so vigilance is important. Pain, failure to progress and a pinkish blue discharge from the post-operative pouch catheter together with a raised C-reactive protein and white blood cell count will be features. A CT with intravenous contrast or a pouchoscopy will be diagnostic. Then what to do? Conservative management is not an option. The valve will stenose and become incontinent. So a difficult decision will have to be made to reoperate and even more to decide the correct course of action. If the patient is well a redo Kock pouch or valve revision will be possible. If the patient is compromised resection of the pouch and an end ileostomy may be necessary, or rarely it may be possible to resect the valve but save the pouch and defunction it pending revision at some further date. All difficult decisions. Fortunately this is a very rare condition.

10.5   Valve Prolapse

The usual cause here is a fascial defect or failure to repair the abdominal wall sufficiently or hitch and secure the pouch to the abdominal wall. The defect can usually be repaired and the afferent ileum returned to the abdominal cavity often done locally without recourse to reopening the abdominal cavity.

10.6   Stoma Stenosis at Skin Level

This is unusual early after surgery and dilatation is the first option.

10.7   Valve Slippage

Not obvious until the post op catheter is withdrawn the patient will be disappointed to find the valve is not completely continent of first gas and then faecal material. It usually occurs during the first three post-operative months. With post-operative swelling, oedema and inflammation it is worth waiting for a period of several weeks before deciding that the situation needs further treatment. A CT with contrast via the pouch stoma or a pouchogram will demonstrate the displaced or slipped valve and an endoscopy will rule out any other causes. If the problems persist then valve revision will be indicated.

10.8   Nipple Valve Fistula

Fistulas can occur anytime after the operation and may arise from the nipple valve, the pouch, or a remote loop of small intestine. The knife-less staples may cause a period of ischaemia and if this is maximal at the staple to efferent limb junction a nipple valve fistula may result. Other causes include sutures through the walls of the valve and tied too tightly, overenthusiastic use of diathermy in scarifying the bowel or the erosion of prosthetic material where it has been used. Rarely undiagnosed Crohn's disease may be to blame. A nipple valve fistula is obviously a cause of incontinence and if it occurs early postoperatively conservative management with more prolonged pouch drainage may be effective in decompressing the pouch and allowing the fistula to close spontaneously.

A more major fistula will need the appropriate management for an enterocutaneous fistula with defining imaging, intravenous nutrition and eventually reoperative surgery. Again complete refashioning of the valve may be necessary.

10.9 Valve Stenosis

This is unusual in the early post-operative period but on occasion despite careful management and the timely removal of the post-operative Kock pouch catheter it may be difficult to reintubate the pouch. The options here are endoscopy with a paediatric gastroscope, passing a guide wire or the use of a tracheal bougie as used for difficult endo tracheal intubations. Radiological screening to help may be necessary. The early post-operative stenosis or oedematous swelling will usually resolve. In the longer term endoscopic balloon dilatation may be effective.

10.10 Volvulus, Herniation and Small Bowel Obstruction

The patient will often have had a division of adhesions during the primary Kock pouch procedure so a recurrence of adhesional problems will not be surprising. But the creation of the pouch and the manoeuvres to place the afferent ileum in the correct position can lead to a volvulus in the immediately afferent ileum or an internal small bowel hernia. A volvulus of the pouch itself can result from inadequate fixation of the pouch to the abdominal wall. A CT with contrast, a CT enteroclysis, or an MR enteroclysis may all be helpful in the difficult case and will identify the patient where conservative management is unlikely to be successful.

10.11 Frequency of Early Post-operative Complications

Since the Kock pouch has been less used with the advent of the pelvic pouch there is little current literature on the frequency of early post op complications. Table 10.1 shows the variation in various published series.

Inflammation of the Kock pouch is unusual and is rare in the immediate post-operative period. Treatment includes topical intra-pouch sulphonamides, steroids, systemic steroids and biologics.

A prolonged period of intubation may be all that is necessary for most of these problems unless the patient has a life-threatening condition. Careful assessment and imaging and timely intervention will give the best chance of pouch preservation and perhaps re-do surgery.

Table 10.1 Complications after a continent Ileostomy

Complication	Incidence %
Bleeding	2–3
Leakage and peritonitis	2–3
Valve necrosis	2–3
Valve prolapse	4–6
Valve slippage	3–25
Fistula	0–10
Stomal stricture	3–10
Complications requiring reoperation	15–25
Pouchitis	1–2

Bibliography

1. Cranley B. The Kock reservoir ileostomy: a review of its development, problems and role in modern surgical practice. Br J Surg. 1983;70(2):94–9.
2. Fasth S, Hultén L. Svaninger G the Kock continent ileostomy: influence of a defunctioning ileostomy and nipple valve stapling on early and late morbidity. Int J Color Dis. 1987;2(2):82–6.
3. Tichenor GA, Orkin BA, Lavery IC. A technique for decompression of the obstructed Kock continent ileostomy. Surg Gynecol Obstet. 1990;170(1):75–6.
4. Lycke KG, Göthlin JH, Jensen JK, Philipson BM. Kock NG comparison between radiologic and endoscopic evaluation of the continent ileostomy reservoir. Scand J Gastroenterol. 1993;28(12):1115–20.
5. Lycke KG, Göthlin JH, Jensen JK, Philipson BM, Kock NG. Radiology of the continent ileostomy reservoir: I. Method of examination and normal findings. Abdom Imaging. 1994;19(2):116–23.
6. Klingler PJ, Neuhauser B, Peer R, Klingler CH, Bodner E. Nipple complication caused by a mesenteric GORE-TEX sling reinforcement in a Kock ileal reservoir: report of a case. Dis Colon Rectum. 2001;44(1):128–30.
7. Lepistö AH, Järvinen HJ. Durability of Kock continent ileostomy. Dis Colon Rectum. 2003;46(7):925–8.
8. Beck DE. Clinical aspects of continent ileostomies. Clin Colon Rectal Surg. 2004;17:57–63.
9. Wasmuth HH, Svinsås M, Tranø G, Rydning A, Endreseth BH, Wibe A. Myrvold HE surgical load and long-term outcome for patients with Kock continent ileostomy. Color Dis. 2007;9(8):713–7. Epub 2007 Sep 3.
10. Beck DE. Continent ileostomy: current status. Clin Colon Rectal Surg. 2008;21(1):62–70. https://doi.org/10.1055/s-2008-1055323.
11. Wasmuth HH, Tranø G, Wibe A, Endreseth BH, Rydning A, Myrvold HE. Failed pelvic pouch substituted by continent ileostomy. Color Dis. 2010;12(7 Online):e109–13. https://doi.org/10.1111/j.1463-1318.2009.01856.x. Epub 2009 Apr 2.
12. Nessar G, Wu JS. Evolution of continent ileostomy. World J Gastroenterol. 2012;18(27):3479–82. https://doi.org/10.3748/wjg.v18.i27.3479.
13. Chen M, Shen B. Endoscopic therapy for Kock pouch strictures in patients with inflammatory bowel disease. Gastrointest Endosc. 2014;80(2):353–9. https://doi.org/10.1016/j.gie.2014.03.039. Epub 2014 May 20.
14. Aytac E, Ashburn J, Dietz DW. Is there still a role for continent ileostomy in the surgical treatment of inflammatory bowel disease? Inflamm Bowel Dis. 2014;20(12):2519–25. https://doi.org/10.1097/MIB.0000000000000160.
15. Aytac E, Dietz DW, Ashburn J, Remzi FH. Long-term outcomes after continent ileostomy creation in patients with Crohn's disease. Dis Colon Rectum. 2017;60(5):508–13. https://doi.org/10.1097/DCR.0000000000000815.

Chapter 11
The Role of the Enterostomal Therapist for Patients Operated with a Kock Pouch

Eva Carlsson, Åsa Gustafsson, and Anne-Marie Hallén

11.1 History of Enterostomal Therapy

The cornerstone of enterostomal therapy started with that Rupert B. Turnbull, Jr. invited Norma Gill in 1958, a former patient from the Cleveland Clinic to lead the technical development under his guidance and to provide stoma care service. Both were visionary in their belief that there was a need for specialized nursing care for individuals who had undergone stoma surgery. Surgeons from all over the world attending the program in colorectal surgery at the Cleveland Clinic returned back home and recognized the need for professional and informed holistic care for their patients rendered by a team approach, including a clinical nurse enterostomal therapist. Rupert B. Turnbull Jr. and Norma Gill also started the first enterostomal therapy education in 1961 and many nurses from over the world participated.

Important for the development of enterostomal therapy was the formation of the World Council of Enterostomal Therapists (WCET) in Milan 1978. The WCET is committed to serving the needs of patients and health professionals and is focused on providing a global forum for international debate, discussion and ideas and provides nurses worldwide the access to stoma, wound and continence care specialty education.

E. Carlsson (✉)
Surgical Department Colorectal Unit, Sahlgrenska University Hospital/Östra & Institute of Health and Caring sciences, The Sahlgrenska Academy University of Gothenburg, Gothenburg, Sweden
e-mail: eva.k.carlsson@vgregion.se

Å. Gustafsson
Department of Surgery, Linköping University Hospital, Linköping, Sweden

A.-M. Hallén
Surgical department Sahlgrenska University Hospital/Östra, Gothenburg, Sweden

© Springer Nature Switzerland AG 2019
P. Myrelid, M. Block (eds.), *The Kock Pouch*,
https://doi.org/10.1007/978-3-319-95591-9_11

11.1.1   The Role of the Enterostomal Therapist

Today the enterostomal therapist is a qualified nurse with a specialised education at advanced level. The education provides competence for examination, diagnosis, treatment and follow-up of patients with stoma, continent ileostomies and bowel-operated patients. The enterostomal therapist should work based on a person-centered approach following the patient through the pre-, peri- and post-operative care process during rehabilitation and in the palliative phase. Through the continuous conversation during consultations, the enterostomal therapist have a good knowledge of the patient and his or her needs, views, interests, habits, priorities and roles. This knowledge allows the enterostomal therapist to create conditions for the patient to master the new life situation and support the patient to get the best possible living according to his or her resources and capacity. Being an enterostomal therapist includes to be an educator, consultant, work with complex care situations, development and research as well as being part of a multi-diciplinary team and work in close collaboration with the surgeons.

11.2   The Continent Ileostomy – the Kock Pouch

The continent ileostomy developed by professor Nils G. Kock in 1969 is defined as a surgical procedure that facilitates planned intermittent evacuation of a bowel reservoir through a continent ileostomy with the use of a catheter (Fig. 11.1). The Kock pouch is emptied by inserting a special catheter through the valve 3–5 times per day. The procedure eliminates a protruding stoma, and obviates the need for a stoma

Fig. 11.1 The Kock pouch. (By permission from Professor Leif Hultén)

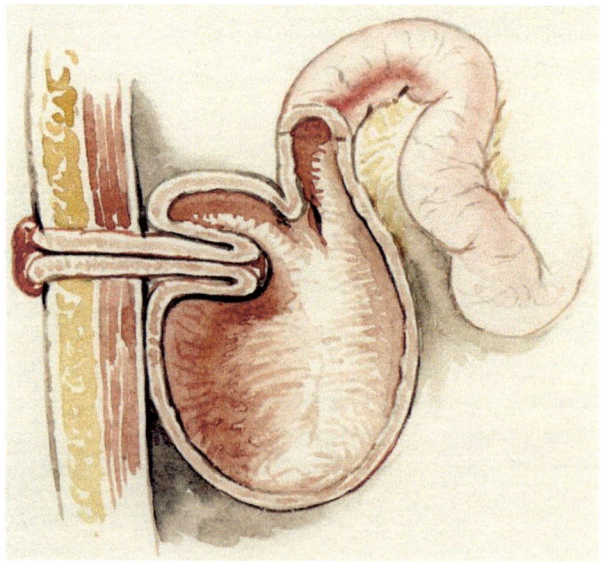

appliance. A stoma cap or gauze square is worn over the stoma. This operation usually involves 10–14 days in hospital.

Most patients who live with a Kock pouch are satisfied with their health status and quality of life and report enhanced self-image, improved self-esteem, freedom regarding clothing, decreased expenses comparing appliances vs. catheters and less sexual inhibitions or psychological embarrassment associated with an external appliance. Negative aspects living with the Kock pouch has been reported to be impediments to bowel evacuation outside of the home due to the quality and availability of public restrooms.

11.2.1   Patients Suited to Be Operated with a Kock Pouch

Today the first choice for surgery for ulcerative colitis is colectomy and ileostomy, and later either an ileorectal anastomosis or an ileoanal pouch. Although the majority of patients with a conventional ileostomy live a near normal life, some patients experience debilitating problems.

Suited for a Kock pouch are:
- Patients who are unsuitable for an ileorectal or pelvic pouch procedure or have poor sphincter control.
- Patients for whom the pelvic pouch has failed.
- Patients who are unhappy with a conventional spouted permanent end-ileostomy and feel that it affects their social life, physical activities and influences body-image and sexual life.
- Patients that have unsolved skin-problems and leakage, hernia, and prolapse associated with their end-ileostomy.

11.2.2   Preoperative Assessment by the Enterostomal Therapist

Patients being considered for a Kock pouch must be extensively counseled about the surgical procedure (pros and cons), the recovery phase (including the first 4 weeks of irrigating, dressing of the pouch and the intubation technique) and possible complications. The patient needs to be prepared that it is a long post-operative phase. If you take time to prepare the patient everything will go smoothly. This is done in co-operation between the surgeon and the enterostomal therapist.

11.2.2.1   Counseling Advice

- Some patients who convert an ileostomy to a Kock pouch have never accepted their ileostomy and are so eager to have a pouch, that they may not at all listen to the pros and cons of the operation
- Tell the patient just to hang in there during the time the pouch is intubated – it is a short period of their life

- You need to describe that handling and caring for the pouch may be perceived as more demanding than having an ileostomy at first. This is because an ileostomy empties in the stoma bag continuously, while having a pouch implies feelings of distension and the emptying of the pouch takes longer than emptying an ileostomy bag.
- It is important with patient education material with pictures for both the patient and the significant other for easier understanding.
- To better understand life with a Kock pouch – meeting other patients is beneficial.
- The importance of keeping a normal weight to prevent complications down the road.

11.2.3   Stoma Siting

Correct preoperative stoma siting has been described as one of the most important factors in the prevention of stoma-related complications and also for the patient's possibility to be self-sufficient in stoma care. One of the advantages with the Kock pouch is that it can be placed further down the abdomen compared with an end-ileostomy since no stoma bag is needed. The location could be approximately 4–5 cm lower than a normal ileostomy and rest on the bony structure of the lower abdomen. Some patients prefer to have it in the same opening as the previous ileostomy. What also needs to be considered is that the patient should have the pouch for the rest of his or her life and therefore should be able to manage the pouch when growing old. Then you need to consider e.g. eyesight, weight gain and it could be easier to intubate the pouch when it is placed higher. The enterostomal therapist and the surgeon need to discuss the pros and cons of the stoma site together with the patient.

On most specialist clinics the enterostomal therapist is responsible for stoma siting, as this is part of their specialist training and is done in consultation with the patient. The patient's wishes should be met as far as possible. When there is a problem with siting or if the siting deviates from the norm there should be a discussion with the colorectal surgeon. The stoma siting is done according to guidelines for normal stoma siting but the ostomy for a Kock pouch can be placed further down. Marking the site for a stoma preoperatively allows the abdomen to be assessed in lying, sitting and standing positions.

- Examine patient's abdomen in various positions (lying, sitting, standing and bending forward) to observe for creases, skinfolds, scars, other stomas, skin turgor and contour. Assess the waist-line, iliac crest, pendulous breasts and the presence of hernia. Observe and discuss with the patient the presence of belts, braces and any other stoma appliances.
- Start with the patient lying on his or her back and identify the rectus muscle. This can be done having the patient do a modified sit up (raise the head up off the bed with knees bent). Placement within the rectus muscle can help to prevent peristomal hernia formation and/or prolapse.

- Choose an area that is visible to the patient. When the patient is in a wheelchair it is most important to consider how the site works in the sitting position.
- If the abdomen is large, choose the apex of the mound or if the patient is extremely obese, site the stoma in the upper abdominal quadrants.
- Mark sites on the right and left sides of the abdomen to prepare for a change in the surgical outcome. An ileostomy and a Kock pouch are normally sited on the right side of the abdomen but there might be contradictions such as a parastomal hernia, skin problems or that the patient prefers to have it on the left side (e.g. dancing, playing the accordion).
- Clean the desired site with alcohol and allow to dry. Mark the selected site with a surgical marker. The mark can be covered with transparent film dressing.
- Make sure that the patient can see the site.

11.2.4 Post-operative Care for Patients with a Kock Pouch

Professor Kock once said that *"While my surgery is important as important is the post-operative care of the pouch because if that fails so does my operation!"*. It is of utmost importance to teach the health care staff of the post-operative monitoring of the pouch. This education is often the responsibility of the enterostomal therapist.

At the end of surgery a curved ileostomy catheter is positioned into the pouch for securing continuous gravity drainage and is fixated by two sutures to the skin (Fig. 11.2). The catheter is connected to a drainage bag and the pouch is continuously drained for 14 days. It is of utmost importance to maintain adequate drainage of the pouch until the suture lines are healed and the intestinal walls forming the valve have adhered firmly. Care must be taken to make sure that the catheter is not dislodged. In order to diminish friction and eliminate possibility of a water siphon effect, the drainage catheter is connected to the bag by means of short wide-bore tube (Fig. 11.3). If the catheter comes out accidentally it must be replaced immediately. During the first 28 days after surgery a special irrigating regime is used (Table 11.1). Absence of drainage or if the patient complains of fullness of the

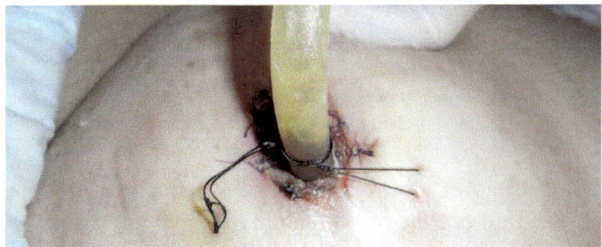

Fig. 11.2 The fixation of the catheter with sutures. (Figures/Photos have been taken by one of the co-authors Anne-Marie Hallén)

Fig. 11.3 The catheter connected to the drainage bag by a short wide-bore tube. (By permission from Professor Leif Hultén)

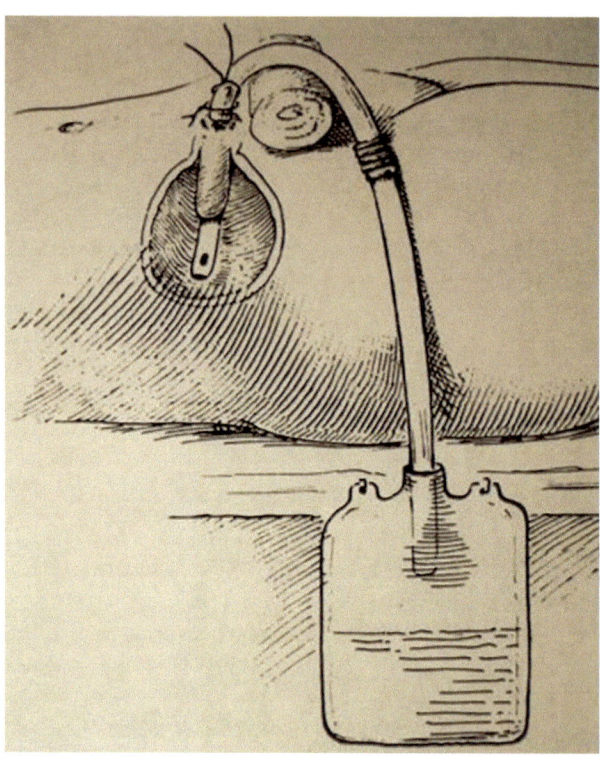

Table 11.1 Post-operative day to day routines - Kock pouch

Day	Routine
First 24 h	The pouch is irrigated every fourth hour.
Day 2–14	The pouch is irrigated every sixth hour and when needed.
Day 1–28	The pouch is dressed twice a day and when needed.
Day 5	The suture that holds the catheter in place is removed.
Day 14	Change the catheter.
Day 14–20	The catheter is plugged during the day and the plug is removed every hour – Pouch irrigated. During night connected to a drainage bag.
Day 21–27	The plug is removed every 2 h – Pouch irrigated.
Day 28	The catheter is removed- at an out patient visit and the patient are trained to intubate the pouch.
Week 5	The pouch is emptied every third hour and once during night.
Finally	The pouch is emptied 3–5 times a day and when necessary and irrigated at least once depending of the consistency of the output.

pouch suggests obstruction. Post-operative pain assessment is important for well-being and mobilization, but the nurse should not give any painkillers until having made sure that the catheter is not blocked. Post-operative high output from the pouch is common for a few days.

11.2.4.1   Irrigating the Kock Pouch

- The irrigating regime for the Kock pouch, is done according to a specially developed schedule (Table 11.1).
- Use portions of 20–30 ml sterile saline for the first 24 h, then use lukewarm tap water.
- Drain the contents of the pouch along with the water that have been inserted.
- Do not withdraw the water that has been inserted or the faecal contents into the syringe.
- At every flushing occasion use between 300 and 500 ml, or until the output is clear and gas is coming. Catheter position and the stoma are monitored each time irrigation is performed.
- If a revision of the pouch or the nipple valve has been re-made, the irrigation solution is increased to portions of 50 ml 2–3 days postoperatively.
- Measure the amount of irrigation solution you insert and what comes out and note on a special chart. If there is a decrease of output (less than you inserted) check if it comes out later.
- Check the catheter frequently once the patient starts eating solid food and ensure that mucus or undigested food does not block the catheter.
- If there is a problem with blockage gently flush until the catheter drains freely, move the catheter slightly or rotate it gently to help clear the catheter, milking the catheter may also help. If it fails notify the surgeon.

11.2.4.2   Stoma Care and Dressing of the Kock Pouch (Figs. 11.4 and 11.5a–e)

- Remove the used dressing.
- Inspect the stoma, it should be moist and red.
- Clean the peristomal skin with tap water.
- Start by fixating the ileostomy catheter vertically with silk tape. Make a pinch under the catheter which prevents pressure (Fig. 11.5a).
- Make sure the catheter is in the middle of the stoma not pressuring against the mucosa.
- Continue with a silk tape and fixate horizontally (Fig.11.5b).
- Start with the tape a bit down on the catheter and drag it across the abdominal incision towards the hip. This secures the catheter.
- Remember not to have a catheter without fixation at any time - the patient can help to keep it in place if you need to change the tape.
- Make a roll of 4–6 non-woven swabs 10 × 10 cm.
- Unfold the outer swab and roll around to hold the roll together.
- Ad the swab roll under the catheter and a non-woven swab around the stoma with its end under the roll (Fig. 11.5c). This swab can then easily be removed without having to change the whole bandage and this also applies for the swab roll since it is not fixated with a tape.

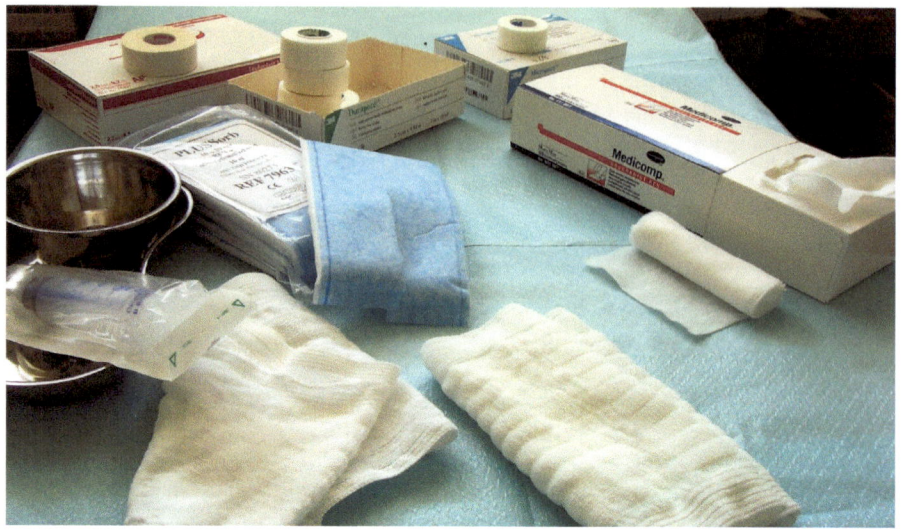

Fig. 11.4 Material used to irrigate and dress the pouch. (Figures/Photos have been taken by one of the co-authors Anne-Marie Hallén)

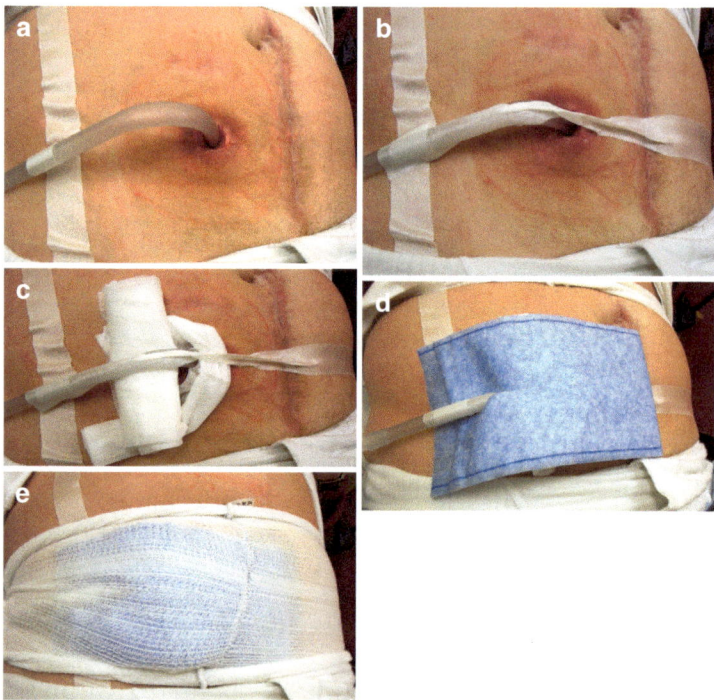

Fig. 11.5 (**a**) Fixation of the catheter vertically. (**b**) Fixation of the catheter horizontally. (**c**) Dressing of the pouch with swab rolls. (**d**) Continue to dress with an absorber pad. (**e**) Net trouser for better fixation. (Figures/Photos have been taken by one of the co-authors Anne-Marie Hallén)

- Cut a notch in the absorber pad and place it around the catheter, fixate if needed with a paper tape (Fig. 11.5d).
- To secure the bandage and the absorption pad, use a net trouser (Fig. 11.5e). This is comfortable for the patient and the catheter is better fixated.

11.2.4.3   Removal of the Catheter and Intubation of the Kock Pouch

On the fifth day of the operation the sutures holding the catheter are cut, and left attached to the catheter as a marker or you mark the position with a waterproof pen. Then the right position of the catheter is known and if it moves out a bit it can be inserted again at the right position. If you remove the old catheter you use the mark on the old catheter to measure out the right position on the new catheter before you put it into the pouch. Some surgical departments have the sutures in place for longer, but we have found this measure advantageous since the catheter can be moved and inserted deeper as the Kock pouch grows larger and it is also less painful for the patient without the sutures.

The patient education focuses on dressing technique, catheter management and the irrigation of the pouch. At first the patient can assist and hold the catheter and then gradually take over the procedure. On day 14, when needed, the old catheter can be changed the education about the intubation technique starts.

11.2.4.4   Intubation of the Kock Pouch and Material Needed (Fig. 11.6)

- The first time the new pouch is intubated, the enterostomal therapist should examine the stoma and the direction of the valve by gently inserting a gloved finger. Then the patient will know in which direction to insert the catheter.
- A curved catheter is used on day 14 if the old catheter is changed to a new, otherwise use a straight catheter 30 French for normal use.
- Water-soluble lubricant.
- Irrigation syringe 50–60 ml.
- Irrigation solution – lukewarm tap water.
- Appliance with absorption pad.
- Peri-stomal skin protection when needed.
- The patient sits on the toilet seat or on a chair beside the toilet (Fig. 11.7a, b).
- Lubricate the catheter with water-soluble lubricant and insert it gently into the stoma and the pouch.
- Advance the catheter through the stoma into the pouch using gentle pressure. A resistance will be felt when the catheter reaches the nipple valve, continue to advance the catheter into the pouch.
- As soon as the catheter is inside the pouch, gas and faecal matter begin to be expelled.

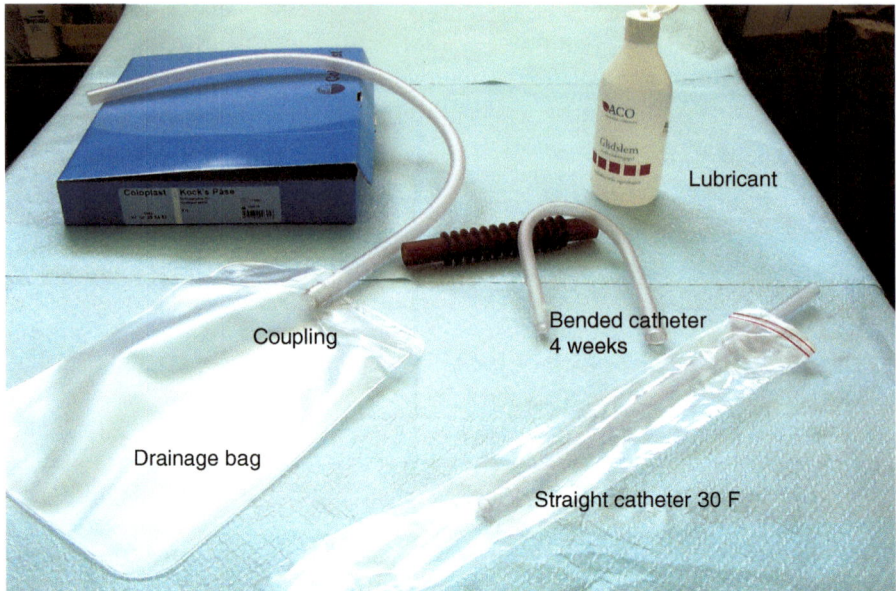

Fig. 11.6 Material needed for intubation of the pouch day 14. (Figures/Photos have been taken by one of the co-authors Anne-Marie Hallén)

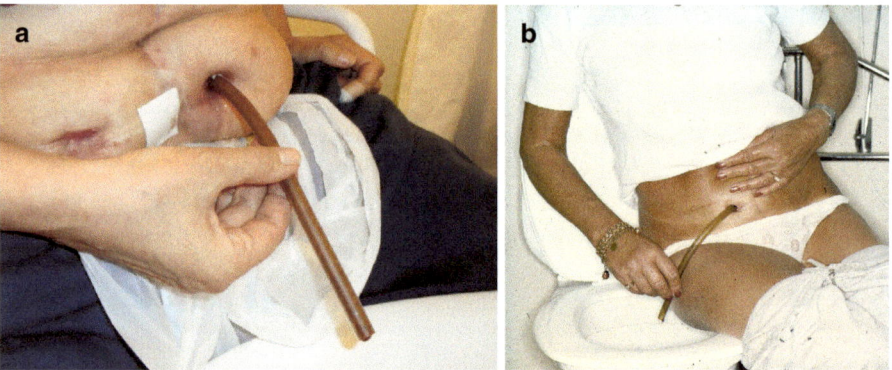

Fig. 11.7 (**a–b**) Patients emptying the Kock pouch. (Figures/Photos have been taken by one of the co-authors Anne-Marie Hallén)

- When drainage has stopped, flush the pouch with the irrigating syringe, 30 ml of tap water (newly constructed) or 50 ml (revision), each time until output is clear and gas is coming.
- Day 14: connect the catheter to a drainage bag. Day 28: remove the catheter smoothly from the pouch.
- Wash through the catheter with mild soap and warm water, then rinse and allow the catheter to dry (from day 28).
- Dress the stoma with an appropriate appliance.

Table 11.2 Post-operative diet restrictions with a Kock pouch while the pouch is connected to a drainage bag – one recommendation

	Pureed ileum reservoir diet (PIR) Day 1–14	Ileum reservoir diet (IR) Day 14–28
Food, in general	Almost all food pureed except for meat (should be minced) and fish.	Food not pureed.
	Not allowed	*Not allowed*
Meat and Fish	Beef stew or fish stew with whole vegetables or root crops.	Beef stew or fish stew with whole vegetables or root crops.
Vegetables and Root crops	Raw whole vegetables and root crops. Boiled whole vegetables and root crops.	Raw vegetables and root crops (peeled tomato and bell peppers allowed). Fried potatoes, french fries.
Fruit and Berries	Raw fruit. Raw and frozen berries. Whole cooked berries. Jam.	Fruit with peel.
Grain products	Whole meal bread, both soft and hard. Rice, pasta, macaroni. Bulgur, couscous, quinoa. Corn.	Whole meal bread, both soft and hard. Rice, pasta, macaroni. Bulgur, couscous, quinoa. Corn.
Other products	Whole nuts, almonds and coconut. Dried fruit.	Whole nuts, almonds and coconut. Dried fruit.
	Other advice	*Other advice*
	Orange wedges should always be avoided. Jam can be replaced with baby food puree or pureed berries.	Orange wedges should always be avoided. Cauliflower and broccoli bouquets should be well-boiled. Fruit must be mature.

11.2.4.5   Diet Requirements

The patient can start to drink and eat on the surgeon's recommendation. There are diet restrictions, especially during the first 4 weeks (Table 11.2). The diet is intended to avoid excess gas, maintain a soft stool and avoid obstruction of the catheter. The patient is instructed to chew the food well at all times.

- During the first 14 days a pureed ileum reservoir diet may be used.
- When the patient starts to plug the catheter she/he may eat an ileum reservoir diet (not pureed).

11.2.5   Preparing for Discharge

The patient will normally stay in hospital for 10–14 days when the pouch is newly constructed and leave on the day when the plugging procedure of the pouch starts (Table 11.1). The patient has a discharge conversation with the surgeon and the

Fig. 11.8 Material needed for intubation of the pouch day 28. (Figures/Photos have been taken by one of the co-authors Anne-Marie Hallén)

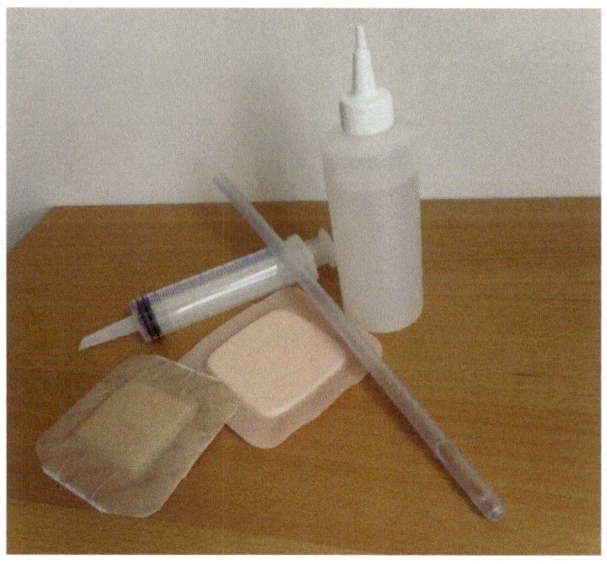

enterostomal therapist and is provided with a written education material of pouch management as well as dietary instructions. All patients with a Kock pouch should have a medic alert identification card or a medical alert bracelet in case of accidental injury and when seeking healthcare. The patient also needs to have stoma equipment for the following 14 days at home to dress and irrigate the pouch. An outpatient visit to an enterostomal therapist is also scheduled on day 28 for removing of the catheter and for education and training to intubate the pouch.

11.2.6 Follow-Up by the Enterostomal Therapist

The patient usually comes on a day visit to the outpatients´ clinic and train the intubation technique (Fig. 11.8). It is done a couple of times with an interval of 2 h (the pouch needs to contain faeces to be easier to intubate) until feeling secure of the procedure.If the patient lives far away one overnight stay could be recommended. Stoma equipment is prescribed and the patients should have the possibility to try out different appliances to find the most suitable. The follow-up may look different, depending on where the patient have their follow up, but usually 2–4 times the first year then by telephone. Patients can also phone whenever needed.

11.3 Pregnancy and Childbirth with a Kock Pouch

The ability for a woman to conceive does not change when she has a Kock pouch and pregnancy as well as delivery should be normal. Just as pregnant women empty their urinary bladders more often, the pouch will need to be emptied more often because the capacity is decreased by the baby's growth. A pregnant woman may find it slightly more difficult to catheterize the pouch during the third trimester, depending on the size of the baby and its position. If this happens it may be necessary to leave the catheter in on free drainage during the third trimester until the baby has been delivered. The woman can have the catheter plugged during the day and empty the pouch at intervals and connect it to a bag during night to have a better sleep, or if she prefers, to have it open during 24 h. If the woman is thinking about becoming pregnant, she should discuss this with her surgeon and her enterostomal therapist.

11.4   Complications-Actions and Treatment

The enterostomal therapist plays an important role in solving and supporting patients with complications either if the patient is awaiting surgery or to solve different problems temporarily for the patient to live as well as possible.

11.4.1   High-Output

When patients have undergone proctocolectomy with construction of an end-ileostomy or a Kock pouch they have lost the absorption capacity of water and sodium that normally takes place in colon. The normal stoma output from an ileostomy is approximately 600–800 ml, but the amount in the Kock pouch is slightly higher. Postoperative high-output (watery) >1500 ml, for a few days, is normal but fluid and water balance must be maintained. Patients with Kock pouch need extensive information about the physiological consequences of high-output, how to prevent it and what to do at home. This information needs to be included in the discharge consultation by the surgeon and the enterostomal therapist both orally and as written patient education material. This can prevent episodes of dehydration leading to reduced kidney function as well as hospital visits.

Actions In hospital: Connect the pouch to a catheter and a drainage bag and dress as described post-operatively. Measure water balance, intake and output (urinary and pouch output), daily weight, blood samples (hemoglobin, sodium, potassium and creatinine). If the high output sustains check sodium and potassium in a 24-h sample of urine. Magnesium may also need to be checked. If the high output occurs postoperatively and sustains, an abscess may be present and then radiology is needed.

Treatment In hospital: Sometimes nil by mouth is necessary, but most often not. The patient should drink unsweetened oral drinks. Every liter of output is substituted with 1 l of parenteral fluid to substitute water and sodium from the pouch. It is important to check for enough urinary output. If the morning weight is reduced from the morning before the fluid substitution is not enough. Medication to reduce ileostomy output (loperamide) is used and taken 30–60 min before meals and in acute situations when needed. When the acute situation is over, replace the intravenous substitution with oral rehydration solutions if necessary.

At home: If this is a normal gastroenteritis the patient may handle this by him- or her-self, but if there is nausea and vomiting involved and the patient is old the patient is recommended to seek acute care. The patient should drink unsweetened solutions, rehydration solution, and increase the loperamide dose. It might also be easier to handle the high output if the pouch is connected to a drainage bag. The patient also needs to observe that there is enough urinary output.

11.4.2 Ileus

Post-operatively or later in life. Symptoms with pain, no output and sometimes vomiting.

Actions Connect the pouch to a catheter and a drainage bag, dress as described postoperatively. Measure water balance, intake and output, see also under high output.

Treatment Radiology and usually conservatively managed but sometimes need of surgery.

11.4.3 Leakage

If there is leakage from the pouch it is not continent for gas and/or faces. The most common cause being slipping of the nipple valve.

Actions Check what type of leakage; gas and/or faces. How much amount of leakage? How often? How often does the patient empty the pouch? Can more frequent emptying reduce the leakage?

Depending on how much leakage, different appliances can be needed; stoma cap when smaller leakage and larger leakage may need a stoma bag. Since the stoma most often is on skin level a convex appliance is often needed to be secure and prevent fecal leakage onto the skin. If the leakage is extensive the catheter may be left in place and connected to a drainage bag. Patients need to be followed by the enterostomal therapist for control of peri-stomal skin and support and the surgeon must be consulted.

Treatment Surgical revision.

11.4.4   Peristomal Skin Problems

Peristomal skin problems in patients with stomas vary and figures between 11% and 45% have been reported. Since a functioning Kock pouch should hold tight for feces and gas there are few problems with skin problems due to fecal irritation. However, the mucous membrane of the stoma can secrete a lot of fluid (moist leakage) which can cause skin problems. The amount of secretion varies and is also dependent of how much the stoma is protruding.

Actions If the patient has a lot of secretion from the stoma use high absorbent dressing to prevent skin problems. If a patient at follow-up presents with skin problems check which pads the patient uses, how and how often he or she changes them. Let the patient try other pads if needed. It is also important to use a new pad (not add gauzes) every time between emptying of the pouch if the patient has a lot of secretion. Extra skin protection, e.g. silicon dressing and/or a barrier cream may be needed. With severe problems, follow-up with extra visits to the enterostomal therapist.

Treatment If the stoma is protruding too much (too much mucosa) it is possible to surgically remove excess of mucous membrane. The best thing is to prevent this at initial construction of the pouch and the stoma.

11.4.5   Fistula

Fistula(s) can occur any time after surgery and may arise from the nipple valve, the Kock pouch, between the pouch and the abdominal wall, or from a remote loop of small bowel. Fistulas that develop at the base of the valve cause incontinence by allowing the fecal stream to bypass the valve. In these situations, the patient will notice incontinence, but will not have difficulty intubating, as is the case with valve slippage. When there is an enterocutaneous fistula the patient will experience leakage onto the skin.

Actions Depending on how large the amount of fistula effluent, different appliances may be needed. Often the patient needs a flange (protects skin) and a stoma bag, which are tried out by the enterostomal therapist. The patient can then empty the bag when needed, but also remove the bag when she or he needs to empty the pouch with the catheter. If the leakage is extensive the catheter may be left in place and connected to a drainage bag. For correct diagnosis an endoscopy of the pouch and radiology is needed.

Treatment Fistulas may respond to drainage, medication or surgical correction.

11.4.6 Pouchitis

Pouchitis is a mucosal inflammation of the pouch. It is manifested clinically by an increase in volume of the effluent and the patient often experience urgency to emptying the pouch more frequently. The content from the pouch becomes watery, foul smelling and sometimes bloody. Patients may also develop abdominal pain, stomach cramps, distension, fever and nausea. The nipple can sometimes be swollen and thus making gas pass through the stoma.

Actions The enterostomal therapist contacts the surgeon to assess the patient's symptoms. The symptoms may be alleviated by catheter drainage to avoid stasis.

Treatment The pouchitis is diagnosed with endoscopy of the pouch and from symptoms. Most people with pouchitis are treated with 10–14 days of antibiotics such as ciprofloxacin and/or metronidazole given orally. Some patients develop relapsing and/or treatment refractory disease and may need long-term treatment. Probiotic bacteria supplements have been found helpful in preventing pouchitis from returning once it has been treated, although more studies are needed. In rare circumstances the pouch may need to be removed. For further details see Chap. 13.

11.4.7 Intubation Difficulties

Intubation difficulties can be acute or developing over time. When the nipple valve cannot be intubated but the pouch remains totally continent, the patient has a functionally complete bowel obstruction and needs urgent medical assistance.

Actions Difficulty with pouch intubation may be eased by relaxing abdominal muscles, lying down on a bed to intubate, lubricating the length of the tube, instilling a small amount of water or air through the tube and if the catheter has been bent to much take a new catheter. It is important not to be stressed, schedule for intubation, empty more often, wait for a while if the catheter does not slide in. A smaller catheter can be used e.g. the same type of catheter for urinary pouch is 24 F. If the difficulties persists it may be easier for the patient to have the pouch connected with a catheter and a drainage bag.

Acute Intubation Difficulties A flexible endoscope can be inserted under direct vision through the stoma into the pouch. Gas and intestinal contents can be suctioned, temporally decompressing the functional obstruction. A guide wire can then be passed through the scope channel and using this as a guide a catheter can be inserted into the pouch to provide long-term drainage and to relieve the functional small bowel obstruction. The catheter should be connected to a drainage bag.

A 10–14 day period of continued drainage may be tried. This provides time for bowel edema to subside and may allow healing or resolution of the problem. If intubation difficulties persist the catheter should remain in the pouch for drainage until the pouch can be revised surgically.

Treatment Endoscopy and often surgical revision.

11.4.8   Stenosis

Skin-level stenosis may aggravate or impair intubation of the pouch. It can result from too small a skin opening at initial construction, intestinal ischemia, infection, healing abnormalities, stomal retraction, and/or repeated trauma.

Actions Several actions may be needed: Try using lidocaine gel when inserting the catheter to reduce pain and use a smaller catheter e.g. a urinary pouch catheter 24 F. A conseal plug could be used as a dilator and be kept in place between emptying of the pouch. The pouch needs to be emptied more frequently. If the stenosis is severe the pouch may need to be drained continuously to a catheter and a drainage bag.

Treatment Often a surgical revision is needed to solve the problem. It can be repaired with a skin level revision or z-plasty repair.

11.4.9   Slippage of the Nipple Valve

Slippage of the nipple valve sometimes occurs in the first 3 months after the operation and is less common after 12 months. Symptoms of valve slippage are incontinence to gas and/or feces and/or difficulty in intubating the pouch.

Actions See under leakage and under intubation difficulties for actions and treatment.

Treatment A surgical revision is usually necessary.

11.4.10   Nipple Prolapse

Valve prolapse occurs when the fascia defect, which is made to bring out the efferent loop, is too large which makes it possible for the nipple valve to protrude through the stoma.

Actions See if it is possible to manipulate the outlet. Use a conseal plug, which may hold the prolapse in place. Try out a two piece appliance, with a stoma bag, see under leakage.

Treatment Endoscopy for diagnosis. Surgical revision is often required.

11.4.11 Other Rare Kock Pouch Complications

- Catheter perforation is a very rare complication that usually requires surgery.
- Dislocation and volvulus of the pouch are caused by inadequate fixation of the reservoir to the abdominal wall. If volvulus occurs, it can result in necrosis of the entire pouch.
- Bezoars, accumulations of foreign material e.g. pills or food in the pouch.

11.4.12 Management Tips

- Draining thick pouch contents may be helped by:
  - diluting the pouch contents with lukewarm tap water
  - drinking two glasses of water, prune or grape juice and waiting a while.
- Teach the patient to only use water soluble lubricant on the catheter. Residues form petroleum gel based compounds may irritate the pouch tissues.
- If the patient is scheduled for surgery where anesthesia is involved the patient should bring a pouch kit to be able to have a continuous drainage of the pouch during surgery, using the same procedure as during the postoperative period.

Bibliography

1. Weakley FL. A historical perspective of stomal construction. J Wound Ostomy Continence Nurs. 1994;21(2):59–75.
2. Stevens P. 35 years of WCET: standing on the shoulder of giants. WCET J. 2008;28(1):8–9.
3. Stevens P. 30 years – the inauguration of the WCET. Milan 1978. 2013;33(2):36–9.
4. Sektionen för stomiterapeuter och sjuksköterskor inom kolorektal omvårdnad (SSKR) & svensk sjuksköterskeförening. Kompetensbeskrivning legitimerad sjuksköterska med specialisering inom stomiterapi, (2017) (Swedish).
5. WCET. In: Zulkowski K, Ayello E, Stelton S, editors. International ostomy guidelines. Perth; 2014.
6. Kock NG. Intra-abdominal "reservoir" in patients with permanent ileostomy. Preliminary observations on a procedure resulting in fecal "continence" in five ileostomy patients. Arch Surg. 1969;99(2):223–31.
7. Kock NG, Myrvold HE, Nilsson LO, Ahren C. Construction of a stable nipple valve for the continent ileostomy. Ann Chir Gynaecol. 1980;69(4):132–43.

8. Crawshaw A, Williams J, Woodhouse F. The Kock pouch reconsidered: an alternative surgical technique. Br J Nurs (Mark Allen Publishing). 2014;23(17):S26–9.
9. Kohler LW, Pemberton JH, Zinsmeister AR, Kelly KA. Quality of life after proctocolectomy. A comparison of Brooke ileostomy, Kock pouch, and ileal pouch-anal anastomosis. Gastroenterology. 1991;101(3):679–84.
10. Berndtsson I, Lindholm E, Ekman I. Thirty years of experience living with a continent ileostomy: bad restrooms-not my reservoir-decide my life. J Wound Ostomy Continence Nurs. 2005;32(5):321–6. quiz 7-8.
11. Aytac E, Ashburn J, Dietz DW. Is there still a role for continent ileostomy in the surgical treatment of inflammatory bowel disease? Inflamm Bowel Dis. 2014;20(12):2519–25.
12. Nastro P, Knowles CH, McGrath A, Heyman B, Porrett TR, Lunniss PJ. Complications of intestinal stomas. Br J Surg. 2010;97(12):1885–9.
13. Person B, Ifargan R, Lachter J, Duek SD, Kluger Y, Assalia A. The impact of preoperative stoma site marking on the incidence of complications, quality of life, and patient's independence. Dis Colon Rectum. 2012;55(7):783–7.
14. Kwiatt M, Kawata M. Avoidance and management of stomal complications. Clin Colon Rectal Surg. 2013;26(2):112–21.
15. Baykara ZG, Demir SG, Karadag A, Harputlu D, Kahraman A, Karadag S, et al. A multicenter, retrospective study to evaluate the effect of preoperative stoma site marking on stomal and peristomal complications. Ostomy Wound Manage. 2014;60(5):16–26.
16. Carlsson E, Fingren J, Hallen AM, Petersen C, Lindholm E. The prevalence of ostomy-related complications 1 year after ostomy surgery: a prospective, descriptive, clinical study. Ostomy Wound Manag. 2016;62(10):34–48.
17. WOCN. A. ASCRS and WOCN joint position statement on the value of preoperative stoma marking for patients undergoing fecal ostomy surgery. J Wound Ostomy Continence Nurs. 2007;34(6):627–8.
18. Svaninger G, Nordgren S, Palselius IR, Fasth S, Hulten L. Sodium and potassium excretion in patients with ileostomies. Eur J Surg Acta Chir. 1991;157(10):601–5.
19. Baker ML, Williams RN, Nightingale JM. Causes and management of a high-output stoma. Color Dis. 2011;13(2):191–7.
20. Messaris E, Sehgal R, Deiling S, Koltun WA, Stewart D, McKenna K, et al. Dehydration is the most common indication for readmission after diverting ileostomy creation. Dis Colon Rectum. 2012;55(2):175–80.
21. Gessler B, Haglind E, Angenete E. A temporary loop ileostomy affects renal function. Int J Color Dis. 2014;29(9):1131–5.
22. Feddern ML, Emmertsen KJ, Laurberg S. Life with a stoma after curative resection for rectal cancer: a population-based cross-sectional study. Color Dis. 2015;17(11):1011–7.
23. Herlufsen P, Olsen AG, Carlsen B, Nybaek H, Karlsmark T, Laursen TN, et al. Study of peristomal skin disorders in patients with permanent stomas. Br J Nurs (Mark Allen Publishing). 2006;15(16):854–62.
24. Beck DE. Continent ileostomy: current status. Clin Colon Rectal Surg. 2008;21(1):62–70.
25. Andersson P, Soderholm JD. Surgery in ulcerative colitis: indication and timing. Dig Dis. 2009;27(3):335–40.
26. Lian L, Fazio V, Shen B. Endoscopic treatment for pill bezoars after continent ileostomy. Dig Liver Dis. 2009;41(7):e26–8.

Chapter 12
Follow Up and Surveillance

Janindra Warusavitarne and Phil Tozer

A Kock Pouch is created, as described in other chapters, in situations where a patient does not want an end-ileostomy and restorative proctocolectomy has either failed or is not appropriate. It allows the patient to have a continent ileostomy which is perceived to be a better alternative than the Brooke ileostomy, for some patients. Patients who opt for the Kock pouch tend to be highly motivated and wish to avoid an end-ileostomy, and may be more likely to notice changes in pouch function.

Standard follow up for any condition aims to allow early detection of frequently occurring or serious events. In this setting standard follow up for the Kock pouch will be based on estimated risks of any particular complication or progression of the underlying disease. Surveillance for complications is not necessary in the Kock pouch for two reasons. Firstly, long-term follow up studies have shown no predictable functional outcomes that may be detected by follow up. Secondly, complications do not represent predictors of pouch failure, and usually these will be reported by patients, prompting any necessary action. Follow-up is therefore based on the underlying disease process.

12.1   Surveillance for Familial Adenomatous Polyposis

Familial Adenomatous Polyposis requires (procto)colectomy to reduce the risk of cancer and in most situations the preferred reconstructive approach is either an ileorectal anastomosis or ileoanal pouch, often with the former preceding the latter to delay the risks of pelvic dissection until after the child-bearing years.

J. Warusavitarne (✉)
St Mark's Hospital and Academic Institute, Harrow, London, UK
e-mail: j.warusavitarne@nhs.net

P. Tozer
Department of Surgery and Cancer, St Mary's Campus, Imperial College, Paddington, London, UK

© Springer Nature Switzerland AG 2019
P. Myrelid, M. Block (eds.), *The Kock Pouch*,
https://doi.org/10.1007/978-3-319-95591-9_12

Nonetheless there are situations where a Kock continent ileostomy is the treatment of choice. Surveillance has to be considered in all three situations. Based on the risk of developing neoplasia in an ileoanal pouch, current recommendations suggest annual surveillance with flexible pouchoscopy. The risk of adenoma formation within the pouch body increases with time and even in the case of a mucosectomy with hand sewn anastomosis the risk of pouch adenomas ranges from 10% to 75%. It is postulated that changes in the ileal microenvironment and mucosa lead to adenoma formation. The risk of cancer in the ileoanal pouch is more frequently related to the rectal cuff remnant, and in this situation the risk of adenoma formation increases.

It is reasonable to assume that the absence of the cuff in the setting of a Kock pouch precludes any cancer risk associated with this. The risk of adenoma formation in the body of the pouch is not well documented, probably because of the low number of Kock pouches that have been created in the presence of Familial Adenomatous Polyposis. In a retrospective study, Tajika et al. examined the risk of adenoma formation in 31 patients with Familial Adenomatous Polyposis, eight of whom had a Kock pouch. In this group the risk of adenoma formation in the Kock pouch was up to 50% with a median follow up of 5 years. This is the largest cohort in the available literature with most descriptions being isolated case reports, summarised in a recent systematic review.

The majority of the polyps are benign, and whilst there have been no reports of cancer arising within a Kock pouch with adenoma formation, there have been a handful of reports of carcinoma within an ileoanal pouch. This may yet be related to Kock pouch numbers. Importantly, there has been no genotype-phenotype correlation to predict the risk of pouch adenoma formation and so there is no reason to assume that adenoma formations should be less likely in the Kock pouch than the ileoanal pouch. On this basis, the best option is for annual pouchoscopy for all patients with a Kock pouch due Familial Adenomatous Polyposis.

Therapeutic options for polyps are not based on any risk prediction model and are based on expert opinion. For polyps greater than 1 cm, endoscopic therapy is the recommended option but it should be performed by a skilled team as the ileal mucosa is thin with a greater risk of perforation.

12.2   Surveillance for Ulcerative Colitis

In patients with an ileoanal pouch in whom there was no dysplasia or malignancy in the resected colon and rectum, there is no recommendation for annual surveillance, as the risk of dysplasia and malignancy is low. Again, in the presence of a cuff and previous dysplasia, cuff surveillance may be appropriate. The risk of dysplasia in the body of the Kock or ileoanal pouch is thought to be low. Herline et al. from the Lahey Clinic evaluated 767 ileoanal pouches with a mean follow up of 8.4 years, and in this cohort only one patient developed low grade dysplasia in the body of the pouch.

However, a meta-analysis of observational studies showed that the presence of dysplasia or cancer prior to formation of the ileoanal pouch is a risk factor for developing dysplasia in the pouch or anal transition zone. The authors suggested surveillance in this group of patients and it is interesting to note that the risk of dysplasia was similar in the pouch body and the transition zone. The current guidelines of the European Crohn's and Colitis Organisation (ECCO) suggest surveillance of the pouch only in these circumstances. Derikx et al. suggest that in the presence of dysplasia the pouch should be surveyed every 2–3 years, annually in the presence of cancer.

The mechanisms associated with pouch dysplasia or cancer are poorly understood. While it may be reasonable to presume that there are genetic drivers to this, such mutations have not been identified. It has been well established that mucosal alterations occur in the body of the pouch irrespective of whether the pouch is associated with an ileoanal anastomosis. Mucosal atrophy and 'colonification' of the mucosa are well described features associated with pouch formation but there is no complete transformation to colonic mucosa. It can be surmised on this basis that there is a risk of pouch neoplasia in patients with previous dysplasia or cancer, and similar surveillance should be recommended to patients with a Kock pouch. Given that there are isolated reports of adenocarcinoma in a Kock pouch, it is probably reasonable to recommend surveillance in high risk individuals.

12.3   Summary of Follow up Recommendations

No overall regular follow up is recommended for patients with a Kock pouch. Routine post-surgical follow up for familiarisation with emptying the pouch should be mandatory and carried out by professionals experienced in educating patients on Kock pouch function, as well as troubleshooting. There should be an appropriate contact person or helpline to aid the patient with a Kock pouch. This approach has been very successful in managing ileoanal pouches and the same principle can be applied to the Kock pouch. As most of these patients are highly motivated, there will usually be a good relationship between the healthcare professional and the patient to ensure that the pouch can be managed appropriately and there is an overall positive impact on the quality of life.

In the presence of Familial Adenomatous Polyposis, annual surveillance with therapeutic endoscopy for lesions greater than 1 cm is recommended, as with ileoanal pouch surveillance, but the low number of Kock pouches for Familial Adenomatous Polyposis means there is inadequate evidence for this to be based on anything other than expert opinion.

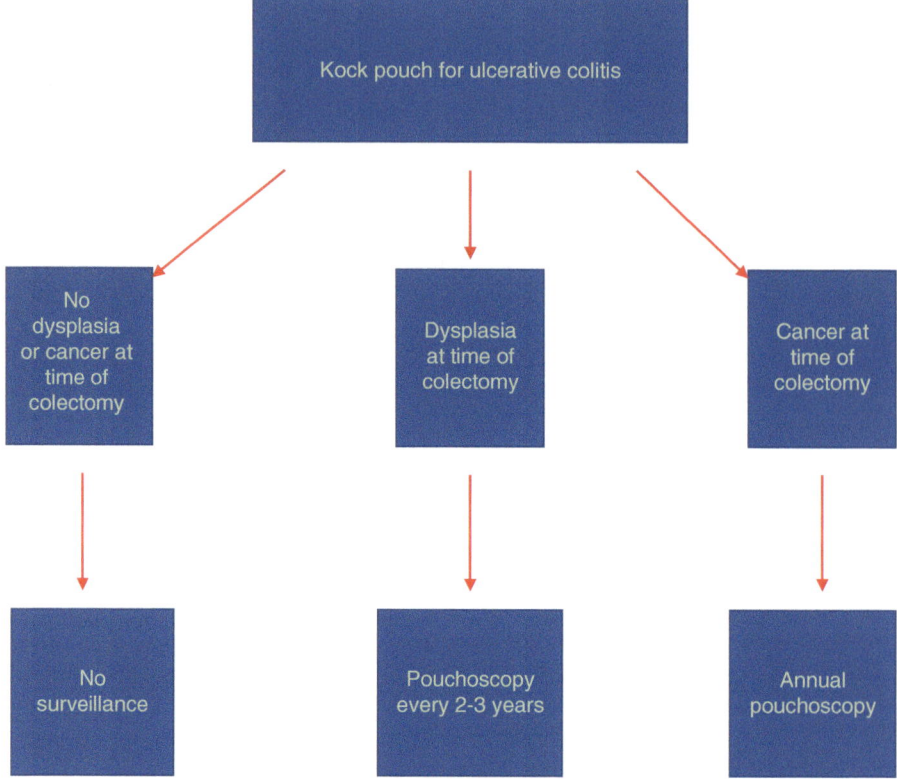

Fig. 12.1 Surveillance recommendations for a Kock pouch created for ulcerative colitis

Figure 12.1 summarises a suggested surveillance regimen for patients with ulcerative colitis.

Follow up and surveillance for the Kock pouch is not based on any firm guidelines owing to the limited worldwide experience of the procedure. The recommendations are broadly extrapolated from experience with the ileoanal pouch. An international registry may be able to shed more light on appropriate surveillance pathways unique to this group of patients.

Chapter 13
Pouchitis

Hagit Tulchinsky

13.1 Introduction

Ulcerative Colitis is one of the two forms of inflammatory bowel disease which violates the integrity of the colonic and rectal mucosa and may have extraintestinal manifestations as well. Along the clinical course of Ulcerative Colitis, up to one-quarter of patients will eventually undergo total proctocolectomy, and about 10% of patients will undergo surgery within 5 years of diagnosis, even in the biological era. The most common indications for total proctocolectomy are chronic active disease despite anti-inflammatory medications, and steroid-dependent disease, commonly designated as refractory inflammation. Some patients undergo surgery for acute severe colitis not responding to rescue medications or when complications, such as toxic megacolon, perforation, or uncontrollable rectal bleeding, occur. Between 10% and 31% of patients are operated for non-refractory indications, among them dysplasia, neoplasia, or strictures. Over the last several decades, proctocolectomy with an ileal pouch-anal anastomosis has evolved into the standard restorative procedure for these patients since it completely removes the diseased colonic mucosa while maintaining normal sphincter function, and avoids the morbidity of a permanent ileostomy. The pelvic pouch is also suitable for most patients with Familial Adenomatous Polyposis syndrome, for patients with indeterminate colitis, and for selected patients with Crohn's disease without small bowel or perianal involvement. Minimally invasive surgery, including laparoscopic and robotic surgery, has recently been applied to pelvic pouch surgery at specialized hospitals, with the aim of minimizing operative scars and possibly improving long-term outcomes. Pelvic pouch surgery has been proven to be safe and effective, with a perioperative mortality rate of <1% and a pouch failure rate of <10%. While a pelvic pouch offers good quality

H. Tulchinsky (✉)
Colorectal Unit, Division of Surgery, Tel-Aviv Sourasky Medical Center, affiliated to the Sackler Faculty of Medicine, Tel-Aviv University, Tel-Aviv, Israel
e-mail: hagitt@tlvmc.gov.il

© Springer Nature Switzerland AG 2019
P. Myrelid, M. Block (eds.), *The Kock Pouch*,
https://doi.org/10.1007/978-3-319-95591-9_13

of life and acceptable long-term functional outcome, it has a substantial rate of complications (up to 60%) that may appear early or late and may be surgical and/or medical, although any clear distinction between them is somewhat artificial. A variety of diseases can affect the ileal pouch, and a correct diagnosis requires a synthesis of clinical, endoscopic, radiographic, and histologic information. Pouch inflammation, "pouchitis", is the most prevalent long-term complication in Ulcerative Colitis patients. Understanding the etiology and risk factors of pouchitis will enable us to alleviate and even prevent it by providing effective treatment to high-risk patients.

13.2 Definition and Classification

Pouchitis is a term that had been introduced in 1977 by Nils G. Kock to describe inflammatory changes in a pouch created from the lower part of the ileum. The term is non-specific, and encompasses a variety of etiologies, pathogenetic pathways, phenotypes and prognoses. Pouchitis may be classified according to etiology, disease duration, activity and responsiveness to antibiotics. It is frequently divided into acute and chronic types. There are two main groups of pouchitis based on etiology, idiopathic and secondary. Based on clinical characteristics of disease behavior, the acute idiopathic pouchitis type is defined as the occurrence of a single inflammatory episode post pelvic pouch creation that responds well to antibiotics and resolves completely after their use. Acute pouchitis might progress to an acute relapsing stage or to chronic pouchitis. Recurrent acute pouchitis is defined as recurrent acute episodes of pouchitis, with up to four flares per year. It is usually antibiotic-dependent, i.e. responds to treatment but recurs when treatment ends. Chronic pouchitis is defined as an active flare lasting for longer than 4 weeks under treatment with antibiotics or anti-inflammatory therapy, or having more than four flares per year. It can be idiopathic or secondary. Based on the responsiveness to antibiotic treatment, chronic pouchitis is sub-classified into antibiotic-responsive, antibiotic-dependent (need for continuous antibiotic treatment to maintain remission) and antibiotic-refractory.

13.3 Incidence

The overall cumulative incidence of pouchitis ranges from 5% to 86%. The variation between different series may be due to the differences in frequency, thoroughness and duration of the follow-up, diagnostic criteria and diagnostic tools (i.e. pouch endoscopy, serial mucosal biopsies), exclusion of Crohn's disease, and the size and the composition of the cohort. Pouchitis is frequently diagnosed within the first year after ileostomy closure, with a reported incidence of 40–70%. Large series from major referral centers reported that the frequency of pouchitis is related to the duration of follow-up, occurring in up to 50% of patients 10 years after. In a recent study, we found that after 25 years post pelvic pouch, 86% of patients developed some form of pouchitis, and that 45.7% gradually developed a form of chronic inflammation of the pouch. Only 14% maintained a normal pouch.

13.4 Etiology and Pathogenesis

Pouchitis is an inflammation that develops de novo in a previously normal ileum that had been used to construct the pouch. The etiology and pathogenesis are not clear, but it is assumed to be driven by an aberrant immune response toward the commensal microbiota in genetically susceptible individuals. The microbiota compositions of patients with inflammatory bowel diseasewere shown to be less diverse and different from those of healthy individuals, an imbalance referred to as "dysbiosis." Intestinal inflammation is associated with alterations in the composition of the enteric microbial population and with a reduction in microbial diversity.Despite an association of inflammation with loss or gain of certain bacterial groups, it is still not clear whether these changes are the cause of inflammation or its outcome. Dysbiosis was also reported in pouch patients, and a long-term prospective study from our pouch clinic demonstrated that decreased microbial diversity per se predicts pouch inflammation.

Recent evidence has suggested that the combination of a decrease in microbial diversity, loss of beneficial bacteria and increase in bacterial groups associated with inflammation contribute to pouchitis. In addition, the altered bowel anatomy promotes fecal stasis in the pouch and chronic metaplasia of the ileal mucosa of the pouch, which could create an environment favorable to inflammation. Examples that support this concept are the absence of pouch inflammation before it is exposed to the fecal stream; the response to antibiotic and probiotic therapies; the correlation of certain microbial groups with disease activity and inflammatory markers; the composition of fecal microbiota in Ulcerative Colitis patients before pouch surgery may be predictive of pouchitis development and the increased likelihood of pouchitis in hosts with a particular gene expression that have an abundance of certain bacteria.

Idiopathic pouchitis is a heterogeneous entity divided into acute and chronic types, both of which are found almost exclusively in Ulcerative Colitis patients. The cumulative incidence of pouchitis in patients with Familial Adenomatous Polyposis is much lower, ranging from 0% to 10%. It remains unknown as to whether acute and chronic pouchitis represent different clinical entities or different spectra of the same disease. The acute type of pouchitis is considered as being a benign self-limited type of inflammation in which patients seem to have distinct characteristics and tend to resemble patients with a normal pouch, whereas the chronic type of pouchitis is an aggressive form of inflammation that causes considerable morbidity requiring long-term multi-drug treatment, repeated endoscopies and substantially compromise quality of life.

13.5   Risk Factors

Various studies that evaluated risk factors for the development of pouchitis combined the acute and chronic types, and relatively few studies focused on either of them individually. Furthermore, data on predictors of outcomes after pouch surgery are conflicting, pointing towards various genetic, histologic, serologic, demographic and clinical markers.

Similar to Crohn's disease and Ulcerative Colitis, there are genetic and serologic markers that have been associated with the development of pouchitis or Crohn's-like disease of the pouch. Some of the markers are associated with a dysregulation of the mucosal immune system, such as the presence of anti-neutrophil cytoplasmatic antibody with perinuclear staining pattern, interleukin-1 receptor antagonist gene polymorphisms and a NOD2/CARD15 gene variant. However, this NOD2 gene variant only exists in about 5% of patients who develop pouchitis and in even fewer patients who do not, and therefore can not serve as a useful predictor. Positive anti-chitobioside carbohydrate antibody (ACCA) serology was found to be a potential marker of pouchitis of any type. A significantly higher prevalence of ACCA positivity was observed in our patients with pouchitis compared to normal pouch patients, with a specificity of 87.5% and a positive predictive value of 83.9%.

The impact of the pre-surgery extent and severity of colonic disease on the clinical course post pouch surgery was extensively studied. Patients who have an extensive disease and/or ileal disease ("backwash ileitis") as well as those with severe disease of the colon appear to be at greater risk for the development of pouchitis. We found that patients with pancolitis were at greater risk to develop chronic pouchitis than those with left-sided colitis. However, some studies found no independent relationship between the extent or severity of disease and the subsequent development of acute or chronic pouchitis. We recently reported that older age at diagnosis of Ulcerative Colitis, older age at pouch surgery, and longer disease duration were associated with a favorable outcome of sustained normal pouch. These differences most likely represent a subgroup of patients with a less aggressive inflammatory phenotype and a lingering course. This also highlights the fact that the surgery itself does not arrest the inflammatory process. An important finding was that a non-refractory indication for surgery (low inflammatory burden) was a distinctive feature among the sustained normal pouch group in which it was 2.5 times more prevalent compared with the pouchitis group. Specifically, approximately 90% and 80% of patients operated for a non-refractory indication, usually cancerous or pre-cancerous lesions, had a sustained favorable outcome after 5 and 10 years from pouch surgery, respectively, while only 70% and 40% of the patients operated due to refractory disease maintained a favorable outcome after 5 and 10 years, respectively [44].

Appendiceal inflammation in the colonic specimen as an independent risk factor to develop pouchitis has been studied in several large series. Our study as well as others did not find any correlation between Ulcerative Colitis appendicitis and chronic pouchitis. However, some studies showed that the presence of superficial fissuring ulcers and active appendicitis were highly associated with pouchitis. The discrepancies between these studies might be attributed to the different grading systems used and to inter-observer variability.

The prognostic role of the occurrence of extra-intestinal manifestations in general, and primary sclerosing cholangitis in particular, which may reflect additional remote inflammation is also a matter of debate. It has been repeatedly implied as a risk factor for chronic pouchitis in many studies but ruled out by others.

The length of follow-up as a risk factor for chronic pouchitis is also a controversial issue. Some authors, including us, reported that the duration of follow-up had a strong influence on the cumulative incidence of chronic pouchitis, while others reported that although it was an independent risk factor for the development of acute pouchitis, no such association was seen for chronic pouchitis.

Gender was found to be significantly associated with the incidence of pouchitis, but, again, there are also data that contradict that finding. A higher likelihood towards males was reported by some authors while others cited a significantly higher incidence of pouchitis among women.

Other reported risk factors are preoperative thrombocytosis, preoperative corticosteroid use, regular use of non-steroidal anti-inflammatory drugs, and being a non-smoker.

13.6   Diagnosis

Pouchitis is an inflammatory process of the pouch and a pivotal factor of morbidity among pouch patients. The common presenting symptoms are non-specific and include lower abdominal pain and tenderness, loose and frequent stools, tenesmus, urgency and soiling. Rectal bleeding, fever, and extra-intestinal manifestations may also be present. These symptoms may be caused by conditions other than pouchitis, therefore it is generally accepted that the diagnosis of pouchitis should be based on clinical signs combined with a typical endoscopic and histological pattern. Because symptoms correlate poorly with both endoscopic and histologic findings, symptoms alone apparently can not be used to identify the presence of inflammation in the pouch. Patients suspected of having pouchitis should undergo pouch endoscopy to verify the presence of inflammation and to obtain mucosal biopsies for histologic confirmation. For optimal histologic evaluation, biopsies should be taken from different locations, including the pre-pouch ileum, pouch body, and rectal cuff. Endoscopic findings include diffuse or patchy erythema, edema, granularity, friability, spontaneous or contact bleeding, loss of vascular pattern, mucous exudates, hemorrhage, erosions, and ulceration. Erosions and/or ulcers along the staple line do not necessarily indicate pouchitis. Histologic findings are acute inflammation, such as polymorphic neutrophil infiltration with crypt abscesses and ulceration, in addition to chronic inflammation, that includes villous atrophy, crypt hyperplasia, and increased numbers of mononuclear cells in the lamina propria. These chronic changes are almost universal and probably reflects an adaptive response of the pouch mucosa to fecal stasis. Until the development of a standardized diagnostic score in 1994, clinicians have used a non-standardized system to diagnose pouchitis. The pouchitis disease activity index (PDAI) is the most commonly used scoring system. It is composed of clinical, endoscopic and histopathologic parameters, each rated on a scale between 1–6, with a total score between 3–18. A cut-off value of 7 is used to differentiate pouchitis (≥7 points) from no pouchitis (<7 points). Several additional scoring systems have subsequently been developed to provide a standardized means of diagnosing pouchitis. The Heidelberg pouchitis activity score (PAS) also combines the scoring of clinical symptoms, endoscopic findings and histologic features. In addition, acute and chronic inflammation are assessed separately in the histologic sub score. The resulting total score (range, 0–36) distinguishes between three grades of pouch inflammation: mild adaptive inflammation (score 4–12), moderate pouchitis (score 13–24), and severe pouchitis (score 25–36). Only individuals with scores of 13 or higher are considered to have pouchitis because some degree of inflammation can be found endoscopically and histologically in almost every pouch, even in the complete absence of clinical symptoms. The modified PDAI (mPDAI) score is derived from the PDAI but it omits histological parameters. In the mPDAI assessment, a cut-off value of five is used to differentiate pouchitis (≥5 points) from no pouchitis (<5 points). Omission of endoscopic biopsy and histology would simplify pouchitis diagnostic criteria, reduce the cost of diagnosis, and avoid delay associated with determining the histology score. Since mPDAI offers sensitivity and specificity similar to PDAI for patients with acute or acute relapsing pouchitis, it might be more suitable for practical use in clinical settings.

13.7   Differential Diagnosis

Approximately 20–30% of patients with chronic antibiotic-refractory pouchitis are mis-classified, and actually have secondary pouchitis. Pouch endoscopy and histology, abdominal and pelvic imaging, serology, stool examination and stool cultures can contribute to the differential diagnoses. It is essential to exclude the following conditions before accepting a diagnosis of chronic pouchitis: secondary pouchitis-like infection, ischemic, drug-induced and autoimmune-associated pouchitis, cuffitis, Crohn's-like disease of the pouch, irritable pouch syndrome, and surgical complications (e.g. occult anastomotic leak that led to chronic pelvic sepsis, and anastomotic stricture). Other less common conditions, such as a small volume pouch, pelvic floor disorders, and pouch volvulus, have to be excluded as well. A normal-appearing mucosa in a symptomatic patient should raise the suspicion of irritable pouch syndrome and other mechanical problems.

Patients who experience pouchitis symptoms immediately post pouch surgery and do not respond to antibiotic therapy should raise the suspicion of surgery-associated complications, such as pouch anastomotic leak. Focal pouch inflammation should also point to the possibility of secondary pouchitis caused by chronic peri-pouch sepsis. A recent study demonstrated that 38% of the patients thought to have antibiotic-dependent or refractory pouchitis actually had chronic peri-pouch sepsis on magnetic resonance imaging studies. Pouch outlet obstruction or anastomotic stricture lead to increased fecal stasis that may result in inflammation of the distal pouch.

An inflamed rectal cuff with a normal or minimally inflamed pouch mucosa in a symptomatic patient should raise the possibility of the diagnosis of cuffitis. Rectal bleeding is a characteristic feature of cuffitis.

Secondary pouchitis due to a number of infectious agents, mainly Cytomegalovirus (CMV) and Clostridium difficile, is infrequent but should be suspected in patients with treatment refractory disease. The clinical presentation and endoscopic features of CMV pouchitis are similar to idiopathic pouchitis with a few notable exceptions. Febrile episodes are more common than the reported prevalence in patients with idiopathic pouchitis. An increase in stool frequency and fever in patients on immune suppression or in those who have failed empiric antibiotics should prompt assessment for CMV infection. The diagnosis relies on the demonstrating CMV inclusion bodies on histology or its antigen on PCR of serum samples. Female gender and immunosuppressive treatments were reported as potential risk factors for CMV pouchitis.

The clinical presentation of pouchitis induced by Clostridium difficile infection is non-specific and resembles idiopathic chronic pouchitis. Therefore, the diagnosis should be based on the combination of the symptoms common in pouchitis, endoscopic findings of mucosal inflammation and detection of toxins A and B by enzyme immunoassay, or toxin B gene by PCR assay in stools. Histologic findings are non-specific and include acute inflammation and villous atrophy. Pouchitis due to Clostridium difficile infection was reported by some authors to be associated with male gender, pre-surgery left-sided colitis, pre-surgery antibiotic use, previous hospitalization, low serum immunoglobulin level and post-operative gastrointestinal complications.

Use of Non-Steroid Anti-Inflammatory Drugs (NSAIDs) is a well-known cause of gastrointestinal damage. The role of NSAIDs use in the exacerbation of inflammatory bowel diseasde is controversial, nevertheless detrimental effects of NSAIDs use on the disease course were reported. Whether the use of NSAIDs contributes to the development of pouchitis is of interest. One study showed that the withdrawal of NSAID use alone resulted in a significant reduction in the PDAI score and a significant improvement in mean quality-of-life scores in patients with a variety of ileal pouch disorders, including chronic refractory pouchitis.

Pouch ischemia may play a role in the pathogenesis of pouchitis.Patients suffering from ischemic pouchitis may have some unique clinical and endoscopic features. Ischemic pouchitis is characterized by an asymmetric distribution of the inflammation in the pouch. The inflammation is typically limited to the distal pouch, with a sharp demarcation of inflamed and non-inflamed parts of the pouch. Common findings on histology are extra-cellular hemosiderin or hematoidin deposits.

Autoimmune-associated chronic antibiotic refractory pouchitis has been proposed in a subset of patients with antibiotic refractory chronic pouchitis, positive serum auto-antibodies (including antinuclear antibody, rheumatoid factor, and antimicrosomal antibody), and concurrent immune-mediated disorders. Increased deep crypt apoptosis is a distinctive histologic feature.

Crohn's-like disease of the pouch is manifested by the presence of symptoms as in chronic pouchitis along with one or more of the following features: pouch-related fistula occurring more than 1 year after ileostomy closure, inflammation of the afferent limb or more proximal small bowel segment(s), or fibrostenotic disease of the pouch.

13.8   Treatment of Pouchitis

13.8.1   Acute Idiopathic Pouchitis

Patients with a first episode of acute pouchitis typically respond rapidly to antibiotic therapy. Metronidazole, ciprofloxacin, tinidazole, and rifaximin have all been used effectively in the treatment of acute pouchitis. First-line therapy includes a 2 week treatment with metronidazole or ciprofloxacin. A few small randomized controlled trials demonstrated that ciprofloxacin was more effective at inducing remission than metronidazole. One study also revealed that adverse effects were observed less frequently in the ciprofloxacin group compared to the metronidazole group. In a randomized, double blind, placebo-controlled pilot study that compared rifaximin and placebo, clinical remission occurred more frequently in patients treated with rifaximin although the difference was not significant. The high-dose probiotic VSL#3 has been reported effective in treating mild acute pouchitis.

13.8.2   Chronic Antibiotic-Dependent Pouchitis

Patients with chronic antibiotic-dependent pouchitis respond to certain therapies but when the treatment is stopped pouchitis relapses, in which case they need to continue therapy in order to alleviate their symptoms. Long-term therapy with various antibiotic combinations appears to be effective. In one small study, ciprofloxacin and rifaximin combination therapy for 2 weeks was reported as being safe and objectively effective in seven of eight patients who either went into remission or improved. In another study, 4 week treatment with a combination of metronidazole and ciprofloxacin was highly effective in 82% of patients with recurrent or refractory pouchitis. It objectively improved the inflammation and patient's quality of life. Another report described sixteen patients with chronic refractory pouchitis who were treated with a 4 week course of ciprofloxacin and tinidazole. The rate of clinical remission and clinical response to the combination was 87.5%.

13.8.3   Chronic Antibiotic-Refractory Pouchitis

Treatment of chronic refractory pouchitis is difficult and largely empirical. These patients do not respond to conventional therapy (combination antibiotic therapy) and often have on-going symptoms. Antibiotic-refractory pouchitis causes significant morbidity and is a common cause of pouch failure, therefore treatment should be relatively aggressive with the aim of pouch preservation. Chronic refractory pouchitis is also associated with financial and economic burdens. There are limited data suggesting the therapy that should be administered in these patients when antibiotic therapy fails. Corticosteroids, 5-ASA, immunomodulators and probiotics have all been tried in clinical trials with either conflicting or disappointing results. The administration of anti-TNF agents has been tried with encouraging results. A systematic review on the use of biologics in pouchitis found that the short-term effectiveness was approximately 80% with infliximab treatment. A recent meta-analysis of 21 papers showed that biologics, including infliximab and adalimumab, significantly induced remission in patients with chronic pouchitis, resulting in a 53% remission rate. Data on vedolizumab for the treatment of chronic pouchitis is limited. There are only a few case reports in the recent literature on the safety and efficacy of using vedolizumab in the management of refractory pouchitis. In one case series of four patients with pouchitis that was refractory to antibiotics and anti-TNF, improved symptoms and measurable improvement in the endoscopic appearance of the pouch were noted after 3 months of vedolizumab therapy.

Fecal microbiota transplantation (FMT) is a novel therapy that involves transferring normal intestinal flora from a healthy donor to a patient with a medical condition potentially caused by dysbiosis. FMT can be performed by nasogastric or nasoduodenal tube, colonoscope, enema, or capsule. There are only two case series and a few case reports that were recently published on chronic antibiotic refractory pouchitis treated with FMT. One study on eight patients treated with FMT via a single nasogastric administration reported variable shifts in faecal and mucosal microbiota composition and, in some patients, changes in proportional abundance of species suggestive of a "healthier" pouch microbiota. However, there were no significant FMT-induced metabolic or immunological changes, or beneficial clinical response. The other study showed beneficial effects of repeated FMT administrations into the jejunum during upper gastrointestinal tract endoscopy: remission was observed in three of the five FMT-treated patients.

13.9 Primary Prevention of Pouchitis

The use of a highly concentrated mixture of probiotic bacterial strains, such as VSL#3, in pouch patients operated for Ulcerative Colitis, was shown to be effective in the prevention of the onset of pouchitis during the first year after surgery and to significantly improve the quality of life of these patients. The administration of Lactobacillus rhamnosus GG was also shown to be effective in primary prophylaxis. The rationale for using probiotics in Ulcerative Colitis patients post pouch surgery is based on substantial evidence that associates intestinal bacteria to the pathogenesis of Crohn's disease, Ulcerative Colitis, and pouchitis. Several mechanisms have been proposed to account for the action of probiotics. These may include modulation of microbiota, enhancement of barrier function, and immunomodulation through direct effects of probiotic bacteria on different immune and epithelial cell types.

Patients with pouchitis reportedly consume significantly fewer servings of fruit and antioxidants compared to patients with normal pouches, possibly exposing them to inflammatory and oxidative stress. The authors suggested that an increase in the consumption of fruits and vegetables, as well as supplementation with specific vitamins, minerals and antioxidants may be beneficial for patients with pouchitis.

13.10   Maintenance of Remission

Relapse or recurrence of pouchitis is common (60%) after completing the antibiotic treatment, and some patients will eventually develop an antibiotic-refractory disease. The first double-blind, placebo-controlled study on the effectiveness of VSL#3 in the maintenance of antibiotic-induced remission in patients with refractory pouchitis reported that long-term administration (9 month) of VSL#3 was effective in maintaining remission in 85% of treated patients. A subsequent double-blind, placebo-controlled study reported similar results. After 1 year of treatment, 85% of those in the VSL#3 group were in remission versus only 6% of those in the placebo group. However, an other study failed to confirm this beneficial effect of VSL#3. In another study, rifaximin alone was reported to effectively maintain remission during long-term therapy.

13.11   Conclusion

The most frequent long-term complication of pouch surgery in Ulcerative Colitis patients is inflammation of a previously normal ileum, a condition known as pouchitis, which occurs in up to 80% of patients and is probably an independent clinicopathologic entity among Ulcerative Colitis patients. The etiology and pathogenesis of pouchitis most likely involves an abnormal interaction between microbial dysbiosis in the ileal pouch and altered immunity in a genetically susceptible host. Pouchitis represents a spectrum of diseases, from an acute antibiotic-responsive type to a chronic antibiotic-refractory. Between 20% and 38% of the patients diagnosed with pouchitis have chronic inflammation which requires long-term courses of antibiotics and/or other medications. Chronic pouchitis may become refractory to medical treatment, causing considerable morbidity with frequent outpatient clinic visits, hospital admissions, endoscopies and corrective surgeries, and possibly ultimately leading to surgical resection or permanent loss of function of the pouch. Moreover, it reduces the patients' quality of life and their satisfaction from the operation. Advanced characterization of patients with Ulcerative Colitis based on combined clinical, microbial, genetic and molecular (expression) variables, both at the time of surgery and after surgery, along with understanding of the etiology and risk factors of chronic pouchitis are needed to develop an optimal predictive tool and to enable prevention of the condition by providing effective treatment to high-risk patients. Given that pouch surgery is inevitable in many cases, and knowing that chronic forms of pouchitis are complex and difficult to treat, early preventive measures implemented postoperatively, such as the early use of probiotics or antibiotics or, in specific cases, immunomodulatory/biological therapy could be suggested to these patients.

Bibliography

1. Allison J, Herrinton LJ, Liu L, Yu J, Lowder J. Natural history of severe ulcerative colitis in a community-based health plan. Clin Gastroenterol Hepatol. 2008;6:999–1003. https://doi.org/10.1016/j.cgh.2008.05.022.
2. Jarnerot G, Rolny P, Sandberg-Gertzen H. Intensive intravenous treatment of ulcerative colitis. Gastroenterology. 1985;89:1005–13.
3. Langholz E, Munkholm P, Davidsen M, Nielsen OH, Binder V. Changes in extent of ulcerative colitis: a study on the course and prognostic factors. Scand J Gastroenterol. 1996;31:260–6.
4. Solberg IC, Lygren I, Jahnsen J, Aadland E, Høie O, Cvancarova M, et al. Clinical course during the first 10 years of ulcerative colitis: results from a population-based inception cohort (IBSEN study). Scand J Gastroenterol. 2009;44:431–40. https://doi.org/10.1080/00365520802600961.
5. Langholz E, Munkholm P, Davidsen M, Binder V. Course of ulcerative colitis: analysis of changes in disease activity over years. Gastroenterology. 1994;107:3–11.
6. Bohl JL, Sobba K. Indications and options for surgery in ulcerative colitis. Surg Clin North Am. 2015;95:1211–32., vi. https://doi.org/10.1016/j.suc.2015.07.003.
7. Van Assche G, Vermeire S, Rutgeerts P. Management of acute severe ulcerative colitis. Gut. 2011;60:130–3. https://doi.org/10.1136/gut.2009.192765.
8. Andersson P, Soderholm JD. Surgery in ulcerative colitis: indication and timing. Dig Dis. 2009;27:335–40. https://doi.org/10.1159/000228570.
9. Nicholls RJ. Review article: ulcerative colitis –surgical indications and treatment. Aliment Pharmacol Ther. 2002;16(suppl 4):25–8.
10. Dayan B, Turner D. Role of surgery in severe ulcerative colitis in the era of medical rescue therapy. World J Gastroenterol. 2012;18:3833–8. https://doi.org/10.3748/wjg.v18.i29.3833.
11. Hashavia E, Dotan I, Rabau M, Klausner JM, Halpern Z, Tulchinsky H. Risk factors for chronic pouchitis after ileal pouch-anal anastomosis: a prospective cohort study. Color Dis. 2012;14:1365–71. https://doi.org/10.1111/j.1463-1318.2012.02993.x.
12. Kaplan GG, Seow CH, Ghosh S, Molodecky N, Rezaie A, Moran GW, et al. Decreasing colectomy rates for ulcerative colitis: a population-based time trend study. Am J Gastroenterol. 2012;107:1879–87. https://doi.org/10.1038/ajg.2012.333.
13. Longo WE, Virgo KS, Bahadursingh AN, Johnson FE. Patterns of disease and surgical treatment among United States veterans more than 50 years of age with ulcerative colitis. Am J Surg. 2003;186:514–8.
14. Wexner SD, Wong WD, Rothenberger DA, Goldberg SM. The ileoanal reservoir. Am J Surg. 1990;159:178–83.
15. Melville DM, Ritchie JK, Nicholls RJ, Hawley PR. Surgery for ulcerative colitis in the era of the pouch: the St Mark's hospital experience. Gut. 1994;35:1076–80.
16. Williams NS. Restorative proctocolectomy is the first choice elective surgical treatment for ulcerative colitis. Br J Surg. 1989;76:1109–10.
17. Fazio VW, Ziv Y, Curch JM, et al. Ileal pouch-anal anastomoses complications and function in 1005 patients. Ann Surg. 1995;222:120–7.
18. Meagher AP, Farouk R, Dozois RR, et al. J ileal pouch-anal anastomosis for chronic ulcerative colitis: complications and long-term outcome in 1310 patients. Br J Surg. 1998;85:800–3.
19. Michelassi F, Lee J, Rubin M, Fichera A, Kasza K, Karrison T, et al. Long-term functional results after ileal pouch anal restorative proctocolectomy for ulcerative colitis: a prospective observational study. Ann Surg. 2003;238:433–41.

20. Muir AJ, Edwards LJ, Sanders LL, Bollinger RR, Koruda MJ, Bachwich DR, et al. A prospective evaluation of health-related quality of life after ileal pouch anal anastomosis for ulcerative colitis. Am J Gastroenterol. 2001;96:1480–5.
21. Tulchinsky H, Dotan I, Halpern Z, Klausner JM, Rabau M. A longitudinal study of quality of life and functional outcome of ulcerative colitis patients after proctocolectomy with ileal pouch anal anastomosis. Dis Colon Rectum. 2010;53:866–73. https://doi.org/10.1007/DCR.0b013e3181d98d66.
22. Fazio VW, O'Riordain MG, Lavery IC, Church JM, Lau P, Strong SA, et al. Long term functional outcome and quality of life after stapled restorative proctocolectomy. Ann Surg. 1999;230:575–84.
23. Tulchinsky H, Hawley PR, Nicholls J. Long-term failure after restorative proctocolectomy for ulcerative colitis. Ann Surg. 2003;238:229–34.
24. Hata K, Kazama S, Nozawa H, Kawai K, Kiyomatsu T, Tanaka J, et al. Laparoscopic surgery for ulcerative colitis: a review of the literature. Surg Today. 2015;45:933–8. https://doi.org/10.1007/s00595-014-1053-7.
25. Homma S, Kawamata F, Shibasaki S, Kawamura H, Takahashi N, Taketomi A. Does reduced-port laparoscopic surgery for medically uncontrolled ulcerative colitis do more harm than good? Asian J Endosc Surg. 2016;9:24–31. https://doi.org/10.1111/ases.12250.
26. Miller AT, Berian JR, Rubin M, Hurst RD, Fichera A, Umanskiy K. Robotic-assisted proctectomy for inflammatory bowel disease: a case-matched comparison of laparoscopic and robotic technique. J Gastrointest Surg. 2012;16:587–94. https://doi.org/10.1007/s11605-011-1692-6.
27. Germain A, de Buck van Overstraeten A, Wolthuis A, Ferrante M, Vermeire S, et al. Outcome of restorative proctocolectomy with ileo-anal pouch for ulcerative colitis: effect of changes in clinical practice. Color Dis. 2017; https://doi.org/10.1111/codi.13948.
28. Buskens CJ, Sahami S, Tanis PJ, Bemelman WA. The potential benefits and disadvantages of laparoscopic surgery for ulcerative colitis: a review of current evidence. Best Pract Res Clin Gastroenterol. 2014;28:19–27. https://doi.org/10.1016/j.bpg.2013.11.007.
29. Shen B, Achkar JP, Lashner BA, Ormsby AH, Remzi FH, Bevins CL, et al. Endoscopic and histologic evaluation together with symptom assessment are required to diagnose pouchitis. Gastroenterology. 2001;121:261–7.
30. Fazio VW, Kiran RP, Remzi FH, Coffey JC, Heneghan HM, Kirat HT, et al. Ileal pouch anal anastomosis: analysis of outcome and quality of life in 3707 patients. Ann Surg. 2013;257:679–85. https://doi.org/10.1097/SLA.0b013e31827d99a2.
31. Mahadevan U, Sandborn WJ. Diagnosis and management of pouchitis. Gastroenterology. 2003;124:1636–50.
32. Shen B, Fazio VW, Remzi FH, Brzezinski A, Bennett AE, Lopez R, et al. Risk factors for diseases of ileal pouch-anal anastomosis after restorative proctocolectomy for ulcerative colitis. Clin Gastroenterol Hepatol. 2006;4:81–9. quiz 2-3.
33. Gionchetti P, Rizzello F, Helwig U, Venturi A, Lammers KM, Brigidi P, et al. Prophylaxis of pouchitis onset with probiotic therapy: a double-blind placebo controlled trial. Gastroenterology. 2003;124:1202–9.
34. Abdelrazeq AS, Kandiyil N, Botterill ID, Lund JN, Reynolds JR, Holdsworth PJ, et al. Predictors for acute and chronic pouchitis following restorative proctocolectomy for ulcerative colitis. Color Dis. 2008;10:805–13.
35. Hurst RD, Molinari M, Chung TP, Rubin M, Michelassi F. Prospective study of the incidence, timing and treatment of pouchitis in 104 consecutive patients after restorative proctocolectomy. Arch Surg. 1996;131:497–500.
36. Tulchinsky H, Dotan I, Alper A, Brazowski E, Klausner JM, Halpern Z, et al. Comprehensive pouch clinic concept for follow-up of patients after ileal pouch anal anastomosis: report of 3 years' experience in a tertiary referral center. Inflamm Bowel Dis. 2008;14:1125–32. https://doi.org/10.1002/ibd.20430.
37. Penna C, Dozois R, Tremaine W, Sandborn W, Larusso N, Schleck C, et al. Pouchitis after ileal pouch-anal anastomosis for ulcerative colitis occurs with increased frequency in patients with associated primary sclerosing cholangitis. Gut. 1996;38:234–9.

38. Shen B, Fazio VW, Remzi FH, Lashner BA. Clinical approach to diseases of ileal pouch-anal anastomosis. Am J Gastroenterol. 2005;100:2796–807.
39. Sandborn WJ. Pouchitis following ileal pouch-anal anastomosis: definition, pathogenesis, and treatment. Gastroenterology. 1994;107:1856–60.
40. Simchuk EJ, Thirlby RC. Risk factors and true incidence of pouchitis in patients after ileal pouch-anal anastomoses. World J Surg. 2000;24:851–6.
41. Shen B, Fazio VW, Remzi FH, Delaney CP, Bennett AE, Achkar JP, et al. Comprehensive evaluation of inflammatory and noninflammatory sequelae of ileal pouch-anal anastomoses. Am J Gastroenterol. 2005;100:93–101.
42. Ståhlberg D, Gullberg K, Liljeqvist L, Hellers G, Löfberg R. Pouchitis following pelvic pouch operation for ulcerative colitis. Incidence, cumulative risk, and risk factors. Dis Colon Rectum. 1996;39:1012–8.
43. Svaninger G, Nordgren S, Oresland T, Hultén L. Incidence and characteristics of pouchitis in the Kock continent ileostomy and the pelvic pouch. Scand J Gastroenterol. 1993;28:695–700.
44. Yanai H, Ben-Shachar S, Mlynarsky L, Godny L, Leshno M, Tulchinsky H, et al. The outcome of ulcerative colitis patients undergoing pouch surgery is determined by pre-surgical factors. Aliment Pharmacol Ther. 2017;46:508–15. https://doi.org/10.1111/apt.14205.
45. Reshef L, Kovacs A, Ofer A, Yahav L, Maharshak N, Keren N, et al. Pouch inflammation is associated with a decrease in specific bacterial taxa. Gastroenterology. 2015;149:718–27. https://doi.org/10.1053/j.gastro.2015.05.041.
46. Qin J, Li R, Raes J, Arumugam M, Burgdorf KS, Manichanh C, et al. A human gut microbial gene catalogue established by metagenomic sequencing. Nature. 2010;464:59–65. https://doi.org/10.1038/nature08821.
47. Manichanh C, Rigottier-Gois L, Bonnaud E, Gloux K, Pelletier E, Frangeul L, et al. Reduced diversity of faecal microbiota in Crohn's disease revealed by a metagenomic approach. Gut. 2006;55:205–11.
48. Gophna U, Sommerfeld K, Gophna S, Doolittle WF, Veldhuyzen Van Zanten SJ. Differences between tissue-associated intestinal microfloras of patients with Crohn's disease and ulcerative colitis. J Clin Microbiol. 2006;44:4136–41.
49. Frank DN, St Amand AL, Feldman RA, Boedeker EC, Harpaz N, Pace NR. Molecular- phylogenetic characterization of microbial community imbalances in human inflammatory bowel diseases. Proc Natl Acad Sci U S A. 2007;104:13780–5.
50. Angriman I, Scarpa M, Castagliuolo I. Relationship between pouch micro- biota and pouchitis following restorative proctocolectomy for ulcerative colitis. World J Gastroenterol. 2014;20:9665–74. https://doi.org/10.3748/wjg.v20.i29.9665. Review.
51. Ott SJ, Musfeldt M, Wenderoth DF, Hampe J, Brant O, Fölsch UR, et al. Reduction in diversity of the colonic mucosa associated bacterial microflora in patients with active inflammatory bowel disease. Gut. 2004;53:685–93.
52. Tannock GW, Lawley B, Munro K, Lay C, Taylor C, Daynes C, et al. Comprehensive analysis of the bacterial content of stool from patients with chronic pouchitis, normal pouches, or familial adenomatous polyposis pouches. Inflamm Bowel Dis. 2012;18:925–34. https://doi.org/10.1002/ibd.21936.
53. McLaughlin SD, Walker AW, Churcher C, Clark SK, Tekkis PP, Johnson MW, et al. The bacteriology of pouchitis: a molecular phylogenetic analysis using 16S rRNA gene cloning and sequencing. Ann Surg. 2010;252:90–8. https://doi.org/10.1097/SLA.0b013e3181e3dc8b.
54. Kuhbacher T, Ott SJ, Helwig U, Mimura T, Rizzello F, Kleessen B, et al. Bacterial and fungal microbiota in relation to probiotic therapy (VSL#3) in pouchitis. Gut. 2006;55:833–41.
55. Maharshak N, Cohen NA, Reshef L, Tulchinsky H, Gophna U, Dotan I. Alterations of enteric microbiota in patients with a normal Ileal pouch are predictive of Pouchitis. J Crohns Colitis. 2017;11:314–20. https://doi.org/10.1093/ecco-jcc/jjw157.
56. Yasueda A, Mizushima T, Nezu R, Sumi R, Tanaka M, Nishimura J, et al. The effect of Clostridium butyricum MIYAIRI on the prevention of pouchitis and alteration of the microbiota profile in patients with ulcerative colitis. Surg Today. 2016;46:939–49. https://doi.org/10.1007/s00595-015-1261-9.

57. Gionchetti P, Calafiore A, Riso D, Liguori G, Calabrese C, Vitali G, et al. The role of antibiotics and probiotics in pouchitis. Ann Gastroenterol. 2012;25:100–5.
58. Machiels K, Sabino J, Vandermosten L, Joossens M, Arijs I, de Bruyn M, et al. Specific members of the predominant gut microbiota predict pouchitis following colectomy and IPAA in UC. Gut. 2017;66:79–88. https://doi.org/10.1136/gutjnl-2015-309398.
59. Morgan XC, Kabakchiev B, Waldron L, Tyler AD, Tickle TL, Milgrom R, et al. Associations between host gene expression, the mucosal microbiome, and clinical outcome in the pelvic pouch of patients with inflammatory bowel disease. Genome Biol. 2015;16:67. https://doi.org/10.1186/s13059-015-0637-x.
60. Penna C, Tiret E, Kartheuser A, Hannoun L, Nordlinger B, Parc R. Function of ileal J pouch-anal anastomosis in patients with familial adenomatous polyposis. Br J Surg. 1993;80:765–7.
61. Tjandra JJ, Fazio VW, Church JM, Oakley JR, Milsom JW, Lavery IC. Similar functional results after restorative proctocolectomy in patients with familial adenomatous polyposis and mucosal ulcerative colitis. Am J Surg. 1993;165:322–5.
62. Dozois RR, Goldberg SM, Rothenberger DA, Utsunomiya J, Nicholls RJ, Cohen Z, et al. Restorative proctocolectomy with ileal reservoir. Int J Color Dis. 1986;1:2–19.
63. Dayton MT, Faught WE, Becker JM, Burt R. Superior results of ileoanal pull through (IAPT) in polyposis coli vs ulcerative colitis patients. J Surg Res. 1992;52:131–4.
64. Lohmuller JL, Pemberton JH, Dozois RR, Ilstrup D, van Heerden J. Pouchitis and extraintestinal manifestations of inflammatory bowel disease after ileal pouch- anal anastomosis. Ann Surg. 1990;211:622–7.
65. Fleshner P, Ippoliti A, Dubinsky M, Ognibene S, Vasiliauskas E, Chelly M, et al. A prospective multivariate analysis of clinical factors associated with pouchitis after ileal pouch-anal anastomosis. Clin Gastroenterol Hepatol. 2007;5:952–8.
66. Turina M, Pennington CJ, Kimberling J, Stromberg AJ, Petras RE, Galandiuk S. Chronic pouchitis after ileal pouch–anal anastomosis for ulcerative colitis: effect on quality of life. J Gastrointest Surg. 2006;10:600–6.
67. Fleshner PR, Vasiliauskas EA, Kam LY, Fleshner NE, Gaiennie J, Abreu-Martin MT, et al. High level perinuclear antineutrophil cytoplasmic antibody [pANCA] in ulcerative colitis patients before colectomy predicts the development of chronic pouchitis after ileal pouch-anal anastomosis. Gut. 2001;49:671–7.
68. Shen B, Lashner B. Can we immunogenotypically and immunophenotypically profile patients who are at risk for pouchitis? Am J Gastroenterol. 2004;99:442–4.
69. Kuisma J, Jarvinen H, Kahri A, Färkkilä M. Factors associated with disease activity of pouchitis after surgery for ulcerative colitis. Scand J Gastroenterol. 2004;39:544–8.
70. Hui T, Landers C, Vasiliauskas E, Abreu M, Dubinsky M, Papadakis KA, et al. Serologic responses in indeterminate colitis patients before ileal pouch-anal anastomosis may determine those at risk for continuous pouch inflammation. Dis Colon Rectum. 2005;48:1254–62.
71. Carter MJ, Di Giovine FS, Cox A, Goodfellow P, Jones S, Shorthouse AJ, et al. The interleukin 1 receptor antagonist gene allele 2 as a predictor of pouchitis following colectomy and IPAA in ulcerative colitis. Gastroenterology. 2001;121:805–11.
72. Brett PM, Yasuda N, Yiannakou JY, Herbst F, Ellis HJ, Vaughan R, et al. Genetic and immunological markers in pouchitis. Eur J Gastroenterol Hepatol. 1996;8:951–5.
73. Aisenberg J, Legnani PE, Nilubol N, Cobrin GM, Ellozy SH, Hegazi RA, et al. Are pANCA, ASCA, or cytokine gene polymorphisms associated with pouchitis? Am J Gastroenterol. 2004;99:432–41.
74. Meier C, Hegazi RA, Aisenberg J, Legnani PE, Nilubol N, Cobrin GM, et al. Innate immune receptor genetic polymorphisms in pouchitis: is NOD2/CARD15 a susceptibility factor? Inflamm Bowel Dis. 2005;11:965–71.
75. Tyler AD, Milgrom R, Stempak JM, Xu W, Brumell JH, Muise AM, et al. The NOD2insC polymorphism is associated with worse outcome following ileal pouch-anal anastomosis for ulcerative colitis. Gut. 2013;62:1433–9. https://doi.org/10.1136/gutjnl-2011-301957.
76. Goren I, Yahav L, Tulchinsky H, Dotan I. Serology of patients with ulcerative colitis after pouch surgery is more comparable with that of patients with Crohn's disease. Inflamm Bowel Dis. 2015;21:2289–95. https://doi.org/10.1097/MIB.0000000000000487.

77. Schmidt CM, Lazenby AJ, Hendrickson RJ, Sitzmann JV. Pre-operative terminal ileal and colonic resection histopathology predicts risk of pouchitis in patients after ileoanal pull-through procedure. Ann Surg. 1998;227:654–62.
78. Achkar JP, Al-Haddad M, Lashner B, Remzi FH, Brzezinski A, Shen B, et al. Differentiating risk factors for acute and chronic pouchitis. Clin Gastroenterol Hepatol. 2005;3:60–6.
79. Lipman JM, Kiran RP, Shen B, Remzi F, Fazio VW. Perioperative factors during ileal pouch-anal anastomosis predict pouchitis. Dis Colon Rectum. 2011;54:311–7. https://doi.org/10.1007/DCR.0b013e3181fded4d.
80. Yantiss RK, Sapp HL, Farraye FA, El-Zammar O, O'Brien MJ, Fruin AB, et al. Histologic predictors of pouchitis in patients with chronic ulcerative colitis. Am J Surg Pathol. 2004;28:999–1006.
81. Dharmaraj R, Dasgupta M, Simpson P, Noe J. Predictors of pouchitis after ileal pouch-anal anastomosis in children. J Pediatr Gastroenterol Nutr. 2016;63:e58–62. https://doi.org/10.1097/MPG.0000000000001279.
82. Samarasekera DN, Stebbing JF, Kettlewell MG, Jewell DP, Mortensen NJ. Outcome of restorative proctocolectomy with ileal reservoir for ulcerative colitis: comparison of distal colitis with more proximal disease. Gut. 1996;38:574–7.
83. Fogt F, Deren JJ, Nusbaum M, Wellmann A, Ross HM. Pouchitis in ulcerative colitis: correlation between predictors from colectomy specimens and clinic-histological features. Eur Surg Res. 2006;38:407–13.
84. Geboes K, Riddell R, Ost A, Jensfelt B, Persson T, Löfberg R. A reproducible grading scale for histological assessment of inflammation in ulcerative colitis. Gut. 2000;47:404–9.
85. Hata K, Watanabe T, Shinozaki M, Nagawa H. Patients with extraintestinal manifestations have a higher risk of developing pouchitis in ulcerative colitis: multivariate analysis. Scand J Gastroenterol. 2003;38:1055–8.
86. Shepherd NA, Hulten L, Tytgat GNJ. Workshop: pouchitis. Int J Color Dis. 1989;4:205–29.
87. Gustavsson S, Weiland LH, Kelly KA. Relationship of backwash ileitis to ileal pouchitis in patients after ileal pouch-anal anastomosis. Dis Colon Rectum. 1987;30:25–8.
88. Hoda KM, Collins JF, Knigge KL, Deveney KE. Predictors of pouchitis after ileal pouch-anal anastomosis: a retrospective review. Dis Colon Rectum. 2008;51:554–60. https://doi.org/10.1007/s10350-008-9194-7.
89. Wu XR, Ashburn J, Remzi FH, Li Y, Fass H, Shen B. Male gender is associated with a high risk for chronic antibiotic-refractory Pouchitis and Ileal pouch anastomotic sinus. J Gastrointest Surg. 2016;20:631–9. https://doi.org/10.1007/s11605-015-2976-z.
90. Joelsson M, Benoni C, Oresland T. Does smoking influence the risk of pouchitis following ileal pouch anal anastomosis for ulcerative colitis? Scand J Gastroenterol. 2006;41:929–33.
91. Setti Carraro P, Talbot IC, Nicholls RJ. Long term appraisal of the histological appearances of the ileal reservoir mucosa after restorative proctocolectomy for ulcerative colitis. Gut. 1994;35:1721–7.
92. Betteridge JD, Armbruster SP, Maydonovitch C, Veerappan GR. Inflammatory bowel disease prevalence by age, gender, race, and geographic location in the U.S. military health care population. Inflamm Bowel Dis. 2013;19:1421–7.
93. Okon A, Dubinsky M, Vasilauskas EA, Papadakis KA, Ippoliti A, Targan SR, et al. Elevated platelet count before ileal pouch–anal anastomosis for ulcerative colitis is associated with the development of chronic pouchitis. Am Surg. 2005;71:821–6.
94. Merrett MN, Mortensen N, Kettlewell M, Jewell DO. Smoking may prevent pouchitis in patients with restorative proctocolectomy for ulcerative colitis. Gut. 1996;38:362–4.
95. Magro F, Gionchetti P, Eliakim R, Ardizzone S, Armuzzi A, Barreiro-De Acosta M, et al. European Crohn's and colitis organisation [ECCO]. Third European evidence-based consensus on diagnosis and Management of Ulcerative Colitis. Part 1: definitions, diagnosis, extra-intestinal manifestations, pregnancy, Cancer surveillance, surgery, and Ileo-anal pouch disorders. J Crohns Colitis. 2017;11:649–70. https://doi.org/10.1093/ecco-jcc/jjx008.
96. Ben-Bassat O, Tyler AD, Xu W, Kirsch R, Schaeffer DF, Walsh J, et al. Ileal pouch symptoms do not correlate with inflammation of the pouch. Clin Gastroenterol Hepatol. 2014;12:831–7. e2. https://doi.org/10.1016/j.cgh.2013.09.027.

97. Tytgat GN, van Deventer SJ. Pouchitis. Int J Color Dis. 1988;3:226–8.
98. Pemberton JH. The problem with pouchitis. Gastroenterology. 1993;104:1209–11.
99. Moskowitz RL, Shepherd NA, Nicholls RJ. An assessment of inflammation in the reservoir after restorative proctocolectomy with ileoanal ileal reservoir. Int J Color Dis. 1986;1:167–74.
100. Shepherd NA, Jass JR, Duval I, Moskowitz RL, Nicholls RJ, Morson BC. Restorative proctocolectomy with ileal reservoir: pathological and histochemical study of mucosal biopsy specimens. J Clin Pathol. 1987;40:601–7.
101. Sandborn WJ, Tremaine WJ, Batts KP, Pemberton JH, Phillips SF. Pouchitis after ileal pouch-anal anastomosis: a Pouchitis disease activity index. Mayo Clin Proc. 1994;69:409–15.
102. Shen B, Achkar JP, Connor JT, Ormsby AH, Remzi FH, Bevins CL, et al. Modified pouchitis disease activity index: a simplified approach to the diagnosis of pouchitis. Dis Colon Rectum. 2003;46:748–53.
103. Shen B, Remzi FH, Lavery IC, Lashner BA, Fazio VW. A proposed classification of ileal pouch disorders and associated complications after restorative proctocolectomy. Clin Gastroenterol Hepatol. 2008;6:145–58. https://doi.org/10.1016/j.cgh.2007.11.006.
104. van der Ploeg VA, Maeda Y, Faiz OD, Hart AL, Clark SK. The prevalence of chronic peripouch sepsis in patients treated for antibiotic-dependent or refractory primary idiopathic pouchitis. Color Dis. 2017;19:827–31. https://doi.org/10.1111/codi.13536.
105. Munoz-Juarez M, Pemberton JH, Sandborn WJ, Tremaine WJ, Dozois RR. Misdiagnosis of specific cytomegalovirus infection of the ileoanal pouch as refractory idiopathic chronic pouchitis: report of two cases. Dis Colon Rectum. 1999;42:117–20.
106. Casadesus D, Tani T, Wakai T, Maruyama S, Iiai T, Okamoto H, et al. Possible role of human cytomegalovirus in pouchitis after proctocolectomy with ileal pouch-anal anastomosis in patients with ulcerative colitis. World J Gastroenterol. 2007;13:1085–9.
107. Shen BO, Jiang ZD, Fazio VW, Remzi FH, Rodriguez L, Bennett AE, et al. Clostridium difficile infection in patients with ileal pouch-anal anastomosis. Clin Gastroenterol Hepatol. 2008;6:782–8. https://doi.org/10.1016/j.cgh.2008.02.021.
108. Man SD, Pitt J, Springall RG, Thillainayagam AV. Clostridium difficile infection - an unusual cause of refractory pouchitis: report of a case. Dis Colon Rectum. 2003;46:267–70.
109. McCurdy JD, Loftus EV Jr, Tremaine WJ, Smyrk TC, Bruining DH, Pardi DS, et al. Cytomegalovirus infection of the ileoanal pouch: clinical characteristics and outcomes. Inflamm Bowel Dis. 2013;19:2394–9. https://doi.org/10.1097/MIB.0b013e3182a52553.
110. Seril DN, Shen B. Clostridium difficile infection in patients with ileal pouches. Am J Gastroenterol. 2014;109:941–7. https://doi.org/10.1038/ajg.2014.22.
111. Seril DN, Ashburn JH, Lian L, Shen B. Risk factors and management of refractory or recurrent clostridium difficile infection in ileal pouch patients. Inflamm Bowel Dis. 2014;20:2226–33. https://doi.org/10.1097/MIB.0000000000000205.
112. Navaneethan U, Shen B. Secondary pouchitis: those with identifiable etiopathogenetic or triggering factors. Am J Gastroenterol. 2010;105:51–64. https://doi.org/10.1038/ajg.2009.530.
113. Shen B, Fazio VW, Remzi FH, Bennett AE, Lopez R, Lavery IC, et al. Effect of withdrawal of nonsteroidal anti-inflammatory drug use on ileal pouch disorders. Dig Dis Sci. 2007;52:3321–8.
114. Kienle P, Weitz J, Reinshagen S, Magener A, Autschbach F, Benner A, et al. Association of decreased perfusion of the ileoanal pouch mucosa with early postoperative pouchitis and local septic complications. Arch Surg. 2001;136:1124–30.
115. Shen B, Plesec TP, Remer E, Kiran P, Remzi FH, Lopez R, et al. Asymmetric endoscopic inflammation of the ileal pouch: a sign of ischemic pouchitis? Inflamm Bowel Dis. 2010;16:836–46. https://doi.org/10.1002/ibd.21129.
116. Jiang W, Goldblum JR, Lopez R, Lian L, Shen B. Increased crypt apoptosis is a feature of autoimmune-associated chronic antibiotic refractory pouchitis. Dis Colon Rectum. 2012;55:549–57. https://doi.org/10.1097/DCR.0b013e31824ab7c6.
117. Isaacs KL, Sandler RS, Abreu M, Picco MF, Hanauer SB, Bickston SJ, et al. Rifaximin for the treatment of active pouchitis: a randomized, double-blind, placebo-controlled pilot study. Inflamm Bowel Dis. 2007;13:1250–5.

118. Shen B, Achkar JP, Lashner BA, Ormsby AH, Remzi FH, Brzezinski A, et al. A randomized clinical trial of ciprofloxacin and metronidazole to treat acute pouchitis. Inflamm Bowel Dis. 2001;7:301–5.
119. Shen B. Acute and chronic pouchitis–pathogenesis, diagnosis and treatment. Nat Rev Gastroenterol Hepatol. 2012;9:323–33. https://doi.org/10.1038/nrgastro.2012.58.
120. Holubar SD, Cima RR, Sandborn WJ, Pardi DS. Treatment and prevention of pouchitis after ileal pouch-anal anastomosis for chronic ulcerative colitis. Cochrane Database Syst Rev. 2010;6:CD001176.
121. Gionchetti P, Rizzello F, Morselli C, Poggioli G, Tambasco R, Calabrese C, et al. High-dose probiotics for the treatment of active pouchitis. Dis Colon Rectum. 2007;50:2075–82.
122. Abdelrazeq AS, Kelly SM, Lund JN, Leveson SH. Rifaximin ciprofloxacin combination therapy is effective in chronic active refractory pouchitis. Color Dis. 2005;7:182–6.
123. Mimura T, Rizzello F, Helwig U, Poggioli G, Schreiber S, Talbot IC, et al. Four week open-label trial of metronidazole and ciprofloxacin for the treatment of recurrent or refractory pouchitis. Aliment Pharmacol Ther. 2002;16:909–17.
124. Shen B, Fazio VW, Remzi FH, Bennett AE, Lopez R, Brzezinski A, et al. Combined ciprofloxacin and tinidazole therapy in the treatment of chronic refractory pouchitis. Dis Colon Rectum. 2007;50:498–508.
125. Sandborn W, Pardi D. Clinical management of pouchitis. Gastroenterology. 2004;127:1809–14.
126. Patel R, Bain I, Youngs D, Keighley M. Cytokine production in pouchitis is similar to that in ulcerative colitis. Dis Colon Rectum. 1995;38:831–7.
127. Viscido A, Habib F, Kohn A, Papi C, Marcheggiano A, Pimpo M, et al. Infliximab in refractory pouchitis complicated by fistulae, following ileo-anal pouch for ulcerative colitis. Aliment Pharmacol Ther. 2003;17:1263–71.
128. Calabrese C, Gionchetti P, Rizzello F, Liguori G, Gabusi V, Tambasco R, et al. Short term treatment with infliximab in chronic refractory pouchitis and ileitis. Aliment Pharmacol Ther. 2008;27:759–64. https://doi.org/10.1111/j.1365-2036.2008.03656.x.
129. Viazis N, Giakoumis M, Koukouratos T, Anastasiou J, Katopodi K, Kechagias G, et al. Long term benefit of one year infliximab administration for the treatment of chronic refractory pouchitis. J Crohns Colitis. 2013;7:e457–60. https://doi.org/10.1016/j.crohns.2013.02.018.
130. Herfarth HH, Long MD, Isaacs KL. Use of biologics in pouchitis: a systematic review. J Clin Gastroenterol. 2015;49:647–54. https://doi.org/10.1097/MCG.0000000000000367.
131. Segal JP, Ding NS, Worley G, Mclaughlin S, Preston S, Faiz OD, et al. Systematic review with meta-analysis: the management of chronic refractory pouchitis with an evidence-based treatment algorithm. Aliment Pharmacol Ther. 2017;45:581–92. https://doi.org/10.1111/apt.13905.
132. Philpott J, Ashburn J, Shen B. Efficacy of Vedolizumab in patients with antibiotic and anti-tumor necrosis alpha refractory pouchitis. Inflamm Bowel Dis. 2017;23:E5–6. https://doi.org/10.1097/MIB.0000000000000992.
133. Coletta M, Paroni M, Caprioli F. Successful treatment with Vedolizumab in a patient with chronic refractory Pouchitis and primary Sclerosing cholangitis. J Crohns Colitis. 2017;11:1507–8. https://doi.org/10.1093/ecco-jcc/jjx090.
134. Mir F, Yousef MH, Partyka EK, Tahan V. Successful treatment of chronic refractory pouchitis with vedolizumab. Int J Color Dis. 2017;32:1517–8. https://doi.org/10.1007/s00384-017-2854-0.
135. Schmid M, Frick JS, Malek N, Goetz M. Successful treatment of pouchitis with Vedolizumab, but not fecal microbiota transfer (FMT), after proctocolectomy in ulcerative colitis. Int J Color Dis. 2017;32:597–8. https://doi.org/10.1007/s00384-017-2761-4.
136. Choi HH, Cho YS. Fecal microbiota transplantation: current applications, effectiveness, and future perspectives. Clin Endosc. 2016;49:257–65. https://doi.org/10.5946/ce.2015.117.
137. Landy J, Walker AW, Li JV, Al-Hassi HO, Ronde E, English NR, et al. Variable alterations of the microbiota, without metabolic or immunological change, following faecal microbiota transplantation in patients with chronic pouchitis. Sci Rep. 2015;5:12955. https://doi.org/10.1038/srep12955.

138. Stallmach A, Lange K, Buening J, Sina C, Vital M, Pieper DH. Fecal microbiota transfer in patients with chronic antibiotic-refractory pouchitis. Am J Gastroenterol. 2016;111:441–3. https://doi.org/10.1038/ajg.2015.436.

139. Fang S, Kraft CS, Dhere T, Srinivasan J, Begley B, Weinstein D, et al. Successful treatment of chronic pouchitis utilizing fecal microbiota transplantation (FMT): a case report. Int J Color Dis. 2016;31:1093–4. https://doi.org/10.1007/s00384-015-2428-y.

140. Gosselink MP, Schouten WR, van Lieshout LM, Hop WC, Laman JD, Ruseler-Van Embden JG. Delay of the first onset of pouchitis by oral intake of the probiotic strain lactobacillus rhamnosus GG. Dis Colon Rectum. 2004;47:876–84.

141. Ng SC, Hart AL, Kamm MA, Stagg AJ, Knight SC. Mechanism of action of probiotics: recent advances. Inflamm Bowel Dis. 2009;15:300–10. https://doi.org/10.1002/ibd.20602.

142. Campieri M, Gionchetti P. Probiotics in inflammatory bowel disease: new insight to pathogenesis or a possible therapeutic alternative? Gastroenterology. 1999;116:1246–9.

143. Shanahan F. Probiotics in inflammatory bowel diseases. Gut. 2001;48:609.

144. Ianco O, Tulchinsky H, Lusthaus M, Ofer A, Santo E, Vaisman N, et al. Diet of patients after pouch surgery may affect pouch inflammation. World J Gastroenterol. 2013;19:6458–64. https://doi.org/10.3748/wjg.v19.i38.6458.

145. Gionchetti P, Rizzello F, Venturi A, Brigidi P, Matteuzzi D, Bazzocchi G, et al. Oral bacteriotherapy as maintenance treatment in patients with chronic pouchitis: a double-blind, placebo-controlled trial. Gastroenterology. 2000;119:305–9.

146. Mimura T, Rizzello F, Helwig U, Poggioli G, Schreiber S, Talbot IC, et al. Once daily high dose probiotic therapy for maintaining remission in recurrent or refractory pouchitis. Gut. 2004;53:108–14.

147. Shen B, Brzezinski A, Fazio VW, Remzi FH, Achkar JP, Bennett AE, et al. Maintenance therapy with a probiotic in antibiotic-dependent pouchitis: experience in clinical practice. Aliment Pharmacol Ther. 2005;22:721–8.

148. Shen B, Remzi FH, Lopez AR, Queener E. Rifaximin for maintenance therapy in antibiotic-dependent pouchitis. BMC Gastroenterol. 2008;8:26. https://doi.org/10.1186/1471-230X-8-26.

Chapter 14
Late Complications

Pär Myrelid and Anton Risto

14.1 Complications of the Nipple Valve

The most common complication requiring revisional surgery is nipple valve slippage. This occurs when the staple lines can no longer hold the intussuscepted intestine of the nipple in place resulting in a gradual shortening of the nipple, in part or circumferential, and in some but not all cases eventually a total eradication of the nipple (Fig. 14.2). Due to the fact that nipple valve slippage is a gradual process over time also the symptoms vary over the course of the nipple slipping. Initially the problem is often difficulties to intubate the pouch. This is because a portion of the bowel that previously constituted the inner aspect of the nipple has moved out to the subcutaneous space, resulting in an angulation of the catheters way in to the pouch. A minor prolapse of the stoma may also be noted at this time. These initial problems are not seen in all cases of valve slipping. If the slipping proceeds and the nipple get shorter the problem will switch from difficulty to catheterize towards incontinence. Incontinence will first occur only at the highest pouch pressures, most often in the morning when the pouch has not been emptied for a long while. When the nipple is all gone the pouch can no longer provide continence at all and it is practically only a really bad end-ileostomy.

When slippage of the valve is suspected a flexible pouch endoscopy should be performed and with an inverted scope the height of the nipple can be assessed determining whether or not valve slipping is present (Figs. 14.1 and 14.2). Most cases of nipple valve slippage require surgical revision with re-stapling of the nipple, which is

P. Myrelid (✉) · A. Risto
Linköping University Hospital, Department of Surgery, Linköping University, Department of Clinical and Experimental Medicine, Linköping, Sweden
e-mail: par.myrelid@liu.se

© Springer Nature Switzerland AG 2019
P. Myrelid, M. Block (eds.), *The Kock Pouch*,
https://doi.org/10.1007/978-3-319-95591-9_14

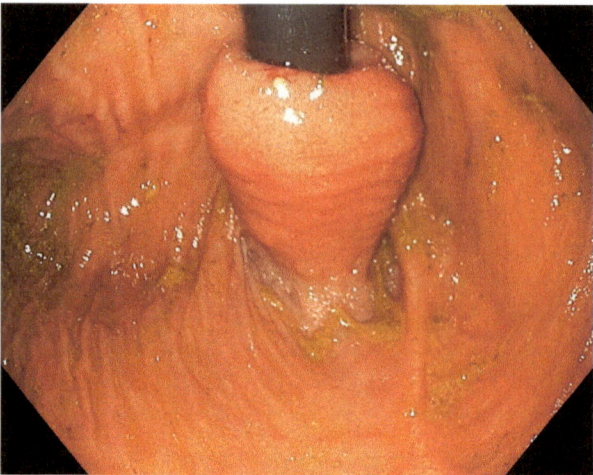

Fig. 14.1 Normal nipple valve seen at endoscopy of the Kock pouch

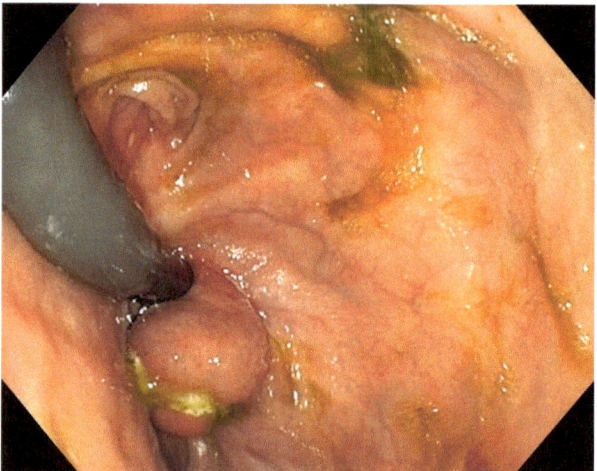

Fig. 14.2 A slipping nipple valve at endoscopy

discussed in detail in Chap. 17. It seems like the risk of nipple valve slippage decreases if the first episode have not presented within the first couple of years from the primary construction but there are several reports of exceptions to such rule as well.

14.2   Intubation Difficulties

The anchoring of the pouch to the abdominal wall is essential to the function of the continent ileostomy. A relatively frequent complication is when this anchoring detaches leaving the pouch hanging only in the efferent limb trough the abdominal wall. This is generally referred to as dislocation or loosening of the pouch. Such dislocation of the pouch seems to be a major risk factor for nipple valve slippage since the two phenomena are often seen together, however both conditions are also seen separately. Dislocation of the pouch can present clinically in different ways depending on how the dislocated pouch falls in the abdomen and if the nipple is intact or not. The most common presentation of dislocation is problems intubating the pouch. If the pouch is still continent this leads to a functional complete small bowel obstruction that needs urgent medical attention. If it is not possible for the surgeon to intubate the pouch with the ordinary pouch catheter the next step is to intubate the pouch under visual control with an endoscope and decompress the pouch by suction trough the scope. It is often possible to intubate the decompressed pouch in the regular manner or over a guide-wire, put in to the pouch trough the endoscope. When a catheter is inserted into the pouch it is advisable to leave it there draining the pouch constantly for some days allowing intestinal edema to subside. In some cases this might even be sufficient treatment and the Kock pouch can function normally after a period of constant drainage. Loosening of the pouch from the abdominal wall can also allow it to rotate over its own axis resulting in volvulus and subsequent bowel obstruction. This will not be resolved by decompression and catheterization. When this is suspected a CT scan should be obtained and if it reveals volvulus of the pouch, the only option is surgery. As mentioned before loosening of the pouch and slipping of the valve often coexist and hence the intubation difficulties and incontinence may well occur simultaneously.

Like all stomas a Kock pouch needs a hole through the abdominal wall which in turn provides a risk that the hole in the fasciae increases in size resulting in a stoma site hernia (Fig. 14.4). In most other instances of stoma site hernia one is not so eager trying to repair it unless it cause an immediate problem such as strangulation of the small bowel. However, in the case of a Kock pouch it is different because stoma site hernia constitutes a severe risk for both nipple valve slippage and pouch dislocation. Because of this it was tried during a period in the 1980s to prevent stoma site hernias by putting in a prophylactic mesh around the stoma when creating a continent ileostomy. It was later shown that this practice to a much larger extent increased development of fistulas than prevented revision requiring hernias, obviously putting a stop to it. Apart from the symptoms associated with secondary nipple valve slippage and pouch dislocation the hernia itself goes, like any other parastomal hernia, with a bulky appearance around the stoma. It may cause trouble intubating the pouch and in rare cases cause incarceration and strangulation of bowel content in the hernia. The diagnosis of stoma site hernia will in most cases be evident with only clinical examination and radiology is rarely needed.

Among the variety of causes for troubles to intubate the Kock pouch a stomal stenosis at the skin level is possibly the most common one. The occurrence of stenosis at the skin level is evident upon ocular and digital examination. The skin stenosis can in some cases be cured with manual dilatation but in most instances local revision of the stoma is required, preferably followed by a period of constant catheterization of the pouch. Once problems with skin stenosis have started they have quite a strong tendency of recurrence. Stenosis of the tip of the nipple valve, or even along the entire length, may also occur and cause problems intubating the pouch.

Stenosis of the nipple is probably due to either relative ischemia of the nipple or fistulas, both causing scaring of the nipple. A too narrow skin opening for the stoma causes problems for the Kock pouch patient but the same holds also for a too wide opening as this may cause the efferent limb to prolapse. If the prolapse is not too great the valve mechanism may still be functioning and the problems for the patient may be limited to secretion from the prolapsed intestinal mucosa and the appearance of the same. In some cases this can be fixed with only a local procedure. A more severe prolapse may however lead to impairment of the valve mechanism with associated incontinence of the pouch. The latter requiring more advanced surgical treatment and sometimes even a rotation of the pouch with creation of a new nipple from the previous inlet. In the case of a strictured nipple valve tip a careful endoscopic balloon dilatation may be attempted but usually a rotation of the pouch is mandated in the long run. The outcome of such revisions is however rather good with up to 94% success rate after one or more revisions.

14.3 Fistulas

With or without meshes fistulas is a relevant problem, in our experience responsible for some 14% of the need for surgical pouch revisions. Fistulas can origin from different parts of the pouch or nipple with the nipple and especially the base of the nipple being most frequent site of origin (Fig. 14.3). This is due to the close proximity to the abdominal wall and that this is where the most foreign material, i.e. sutures and staples are deposited. When the fistulas go from the nipple valve or pouch to the skin they are called enterocutaneous fistulas. These fistulas generally debouch either somewhere near the stoma site or in the scar from the midline incision. There are basically two ways in which enterocutaneous fistulas present. Either if they penetrate all the way through the skin plane which effectively leads to incontinence, not because there is any problem with the valve mechanism, but rather because the intestinal content simply bypasses the valve trough the fistula tract. Before the fistula penetrates the skin it enters into the subcutaneous space resulting in an abscess with palpable fluctuating swelling under the skin and signs of inflammation such as pain, tenderness (especially at time of intubation), redness and fever. These two phenomena may very well occur simultaneously as some parts of an abscess/fistula system may drain itself through the skin while other parts may be entrapped forming an abscess. Just as with the stoma site hernias the presence of fistulas from the pouch to the skin or subcutaneous space are in most cases not difficult to determine with no more than clinical examination, however both pouch endoscopy, CT scan/ MRI, and radiological fistulography can be of value in the planning for optimal treatment of the fistula. Although less frequent than fistulas to the skin or subcutaneous space, fistulas from the pouch can enter into any organ within reasonable proximity, such as other parts of the intestine, urinary bladder or vagina. Fistulas to the urinary bladder present with frequently recurrent urinary tract infections, pneumaturia and intestinal content in the urine. Fistulas to the vagina may cause infections

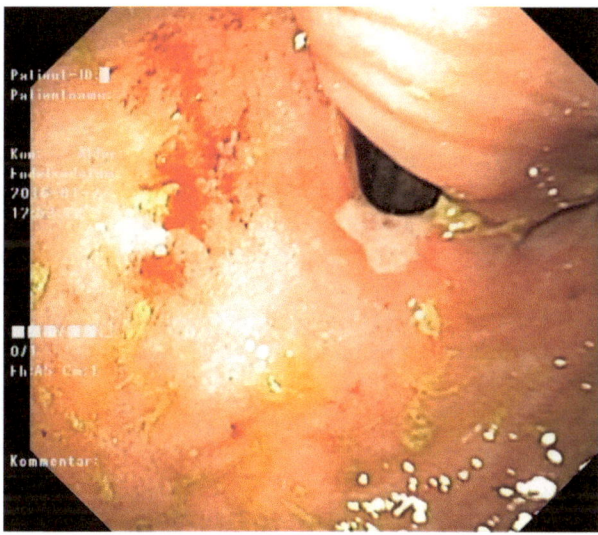

Fig. 14.3 A fistula at the base of the nipple valve causing incontinence. The endoscope is seen through the fistula opening

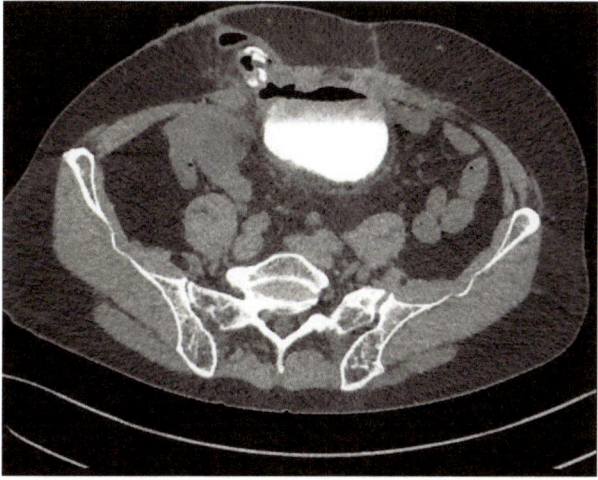

Fig. 14.4 The nipple valve has herniated through the abdominal wall causing intubation difficulties as well as incontinence of the pouch. The staples of the pouch can be seen in the subcutaneous space rather than inside of the abdominal wall on the CT scan

and the passing of gas and intestinal content. Fistulas from ileal pouches can be very hard to remedy and in many patient series, including the one from our own center, it is the most common cause of pouch extirpation and conversion to a permanent end-ileostomy. Still, having that said it does not work the other way around and most fistulas can be cured and the patients can keep their Kock pouches (Fig. 14.4).

14.4 Small Bowel Obstruction

Since the formation of a continent ileostomy is a major intraabdominal surgical procedure, and the vast majority of patients have had at least one abdominal surgery prior to the formation of their Kock pouch, intra-abdominal adhesions are obviously very prevalent in this group of patients. Because of this, small bowel obstruction due toadhesions is more frequent than in the general population. As mentioned above there are also small bowel obstruction causes that are more specific to continent ileostomy, namely volvulus of the pouch due to dislocation or different nipple problems rendering it impossible to intubate the pouch and resulting in functional bowel obstruction. Most of the patients are treated conservatively but surgery may in some cases become necessary.

14.5 Pouchitis

As the name implies pouchitis refers to a general, non-specific inflammation of the ileal pouch reservoir. Just like in ileal pelvic pouches it is very frequent in patients with continent ileostomies and reported in roughly 50% of cases. The clinical presentation of pouchitis is increased volume of ileal content and the content becomes foul smelling, watery and occasionally bloody. Various degrees of abdominal distention or pain, fever and nausea may also occur. Although not completely understood the cause of pouchitis is thought to be, at least in part, bacterial overgrowth since it is usually successfully treated with antibiotics (metronidazol and/or ciprofloxacin). If antibiotics alone is not enough as treatment a period with a continuously draining catheter and/or probiotics might be considered. Treatment is often started solely on clinical findings but for a fully reliable diagnosis pouch endoscopy with biopsies should be performed. Pouchitis is discussed in more detail in Chap. 13.

14.6 Other Problems and Concerns

A concern in the early days of the Kock pouch was that epithelial metaplasia over time could lead to the development of dysplasia and subsequently carcinoma in the pouch. In all published literature on the matter only one such case has been reported and the number in ileoanal pelvic pouches is similarly low and in a national cohort as low as 0.06%. All together this allows us to conclude that such worries where never motivated.

Malabsorption has also been suggested as a possible complication to the creation of a Kock pouch and indeed some investigators have reported cases of severe vitamin B12 malabsorption. However, other investigators have not been able to find such cases and overall it does not appear to be a major issue for the bulk of Kock pouch patients. Moreover, most malabsorption can be successfully handled with substitution medications so if only kept in mind it should pose no problem.

Bibliography

1. Denoya PI, et al. Delayed Kock pouch nipple valve failure: is revision indicated? Dis Colon Rectum. 2008;51(10):1544–7.
2. Beck DE. Clinical aspects of continent ileostomies. Clin Colon Rectal Surg. 2004;17(1):57–63.
3. Beck DE. Continent ileostomy: current status. Clin Colon Rectal Surg. 2008;21(1):62–70.
4. Bloom RJ, et al. A reappraisal of the Kock continent ileostomy in patients with Crohn's disease. Surg Gynecol Obstet. 1986;162(2):105–8.
5. Boostrom SY, et al. Risk of neoplastic change in ileal pouches in familial adenomatous polyposis. J Gastrointest Surg. 2013;17(10):1804–8.
6. Castillo E, et al. Continent ileostomy: current experience. Dis Colon Rectum. 2005;48(6):1263–8.
7. Dozois RR, et al. Improved results with continent ileostomy. Ann Surg. 1980;192(3):319–24.
8. Gerber A, Apt MK, Craig PH. The Kock continent ileostomy. Surg Gynecol Obstet. 1983;156(3):345–50.
9. Giannini I, et al. Adenocarcinoma arising from a long-standing Kock pouch. Int J Color Dis. 2014;29(3):411–2.
10. Henriet MP, Neyra P, Elman B. Kock pouch procedures: continuing experience and evolution in 135 cases. J Urol. 1991;146(1):16–20.
11. Heuschen UA, et al. Adenocarcinoma in the ileal pouch: late risk of cancer after restorative proctocolectomy. Int J Color Dis. 2001;16(2):126–30.
12. Klingler PJ, et al. Nipple complication caused by a mesenteric GORE-TEX sling reinforcement in a Kock ileal reservoir: report of a case. Dis Colon Rectum. 2001;44(1):128–30.
13. Lieskovsky G, Skinner DG, Boyd SD. Complications of the Kock pouch. Urol Clin North Am. 1988;15(2):195–205.
14. Mergener K. Endoscopic management of Kock pouch dysfunction: case report of a method to establish wire-guided pouch access for catheterization. Gastrointest Endosc. 2003;57(6):780–2.
15. Nessar G, Wu JS. Evolution of continent ileostomy. World J Gastroenterol. 2012;18(27):3479–82.
16. Lepisto AH, Jarvinen HJ. Durability of Kock continent ileostomy. Dis Colon Rectum. 2003;46(7):925–8.
17. Litle VR, et al. The continent ileostomy: long-term durability and patient satisfaction. J Gastrointest Surg. 1999;3(6):625–32.
18. Wasmuth HH, Myrvold HE. Durability of ileal pouch-anal anastomosis and continent ileostomy. Dis Colon Rectum. 2009;52(7):1285–9.
19. Wasmuth HH, et al. Surgical load and long-term outcome for patients with Kock continent ileostomy. Color Dis. 2007;9(8):713–7.
20. Agrez MV, Dozois RR, Beahrs OH. Volvulus of the Kock pouch with obstruction and perforation: a case report. Aust N Z J Surg. 1981;51(3):311–3.
21. Svaninger G, et al. Incidence and characteristics of pouchitis in the Kock continent ileostomy and the pelvic pouch. Scand J Gastroenterol. 1993;28(8):695–700.
22. Hashavia E, et al. Risk factors for chronic pouchitis after ileal pouch-anal anastomosis: a prospective cohort study. Color Dis. 2012;14(11):1365–71.
23. Landy J, et al. Etiology of pouchitis. Inflamm Bowel Dis. 2012;18(6):1146–55.
24. Um JW, M'Koma AE. Pouch-related dysplasia and adenocarcinoma following restorative proctocolectomy for ulcerative colitis. Tech Coloproctol. 2011;15(1):7–16.
25. Thompson-Fawcett MW, et al. Risk of dysplasia in long-term ileal pouches and pouches with chronic pouchitis. Gastroenterology. 2001;121(2):275–81.
26. Ståhlberg D, et al. Atrophy and neoplastic transformation of the ileal pouch mucosa in patients with ulcerative colitis and primary sclerosing cholangitis: a case control study. Dis Colon Rectum. 2003;46(6):770–8.
27. Stahlberg D, et al. Atrophy and neoplastic transformation of the ileal pouch mucosa in patients with ulcerative colitis and primary sclerosing cholangitis: a case control study. Dis Colon Rectum. 2003;46(6):770–8.

28. Hulten L, et al. Mucosal assessment for dysplasia and cancer in the ileal pouch mucosa in patients operated on for ulcerative colitis--a 30-year follow-up study. Dis Colon Rectum. 2002;45(4):448–52.
29. Chen KK, et al. Histopathological changes in Kock pouch. Br J Urol. 1993;72(4):433–40.
30. Cox CL, et al. Development of invasive adenocarcinoma in a long-standing Kock continent ileostomy: report of a case. Dis Colon Rectum. 1997;40(4):500–3.
31. Abdalla M, et al. Risk of rectal cancer after colectomy for patients with ulcerative colitis: a national cohort study. Clin Gastroenterol Hepatol. 2017;15(7):1055–1060 e2.
32. Kelley DG, et al. Diarrhoea after continent ileostomy. Gut. 1980;21(8):711–6.
33. Schjonsby H, et al. Stagnant loop syndrome in patients with continent ileostomy (intra-abdominal ileal reservoir). Gut. 1977;18(10):795–9.
34. Jagenburg R, Kock NG, Philipson B. Vitamin B12 absorption in patients with continent ileostomy. Scand J Gastroenterol. 1975;10(2):141–4.
35. Nilsson LO, et al. Absorption studies in patients six to 10 years after construction of ileostomy reservoirs. Gut. 1979;20(6):499–503.
36. Nilsson LO, et al. Vitamin B12 in plasma in patients with continent ileostomy and long observation time. Scand J Gastroenterol. 1984;19(3):369–74.

Chapter 15
Management of de Novo Crohn's Disease after Reconstructive Surgery with Continent Ileostomy in Ulcerative Colitis

Henrik Hjortswang

Pouchitis, i.e. de novo inflammation of the ileal pouch, is a common complication in patients with ileal pouch anal anastomosis (IPAA) or continent ileostomy (Kock pouch) following colectomy for Ulcerative Colitis. It has an endoscopic appearance resembling the colorectal inflammation of Ulcerative Colitis, and causes symptoms with increased stool frequency, urgency, abdominal cramps, mucous and/or bloody exudates, and fever. The cumulative incidence is increasing with time from ileostomy takedown and is reported to affect more than 50% of patients within 10 years and more than 70% after 20 years. For patients who have had one episode of pouchitis two thirds will have recurrent episodes. About 10% develop chronic antibiotic refractory pouchitis.

Some patients with pouchitis develop an inflammation with a phenotype resembling Crohn's disease, although they preoperatively had a clinical presentation, endoscopic features and histopathology data indicating they had Ulcerative Colitis, including reexamination of the pathology specimens. Whether this Crohn's-like condition has the same etiology as Crohn's disease or if it is a new inflammatory entity is unclear. There is no agreed definition of de novo Crohn's disease of the pouch, but it often includes a Crohn-like ulcerative inflammation, involvement of the pre-pouch afferent limb, and non-anastomotic complications with strictures or fistulas unrelated to surgery.

The clinical presentation of this Crohn's-like inflammation can have a wide range depending on the location, severity, and presence of complications to the disease. Most often the symptoms are unspecific and are similar to those seen in other inflammatory and non-inflammatory pouch disorders, such as irritable pouch syndrome, bacterial overgrowth, infectious enteritis, and pouchitis, described above.

H. Hjortswang (✉)
Department of Gastroenterology and Department of Clinical and Experimental Medicine, Linköping University, Linköping, Sweden
e-mail: henrik.hjortswang@regionostergotland.se

© Springer Nature Switzerland AG 2019
P. Myrelid, M. Block (eds.), *The Kock Pouch*,
https://doi.org/10.1007/978-3-319-95591-9_15

15.1 Diagnosis

Making a firm diagnosis of de novo Crohn's disease of the pouch can be challenging since there is no specific marker that accurately can confirm the diagnosis. Instead the diagnosis of Crohn is based on criteria of different disease phenotypes and exclusion of morbidities that may mimic the condition such as infection or other inflammatory conditions. As there is no single way to diagnose Crohn's disease, Lennard-Jones et al. have defined macroscopic and microscopic criteria to establish the diagnosis.

The diagnosis of de novo Crohn's disease of the pouch is thus based on the occurrence of inflammatory bowel changes with a Crohn-like phenotype in a patient reconstructed with an ileal pouch after proctocolectomy for Ulcerative Colitis or indeterminate colitis. Antibiotic-refractory inflammation of the pouch and/or the prepouch ileum with Crohn-like ulcerations or skip lesions, or presence of non-surgery-related fibrotic stricturing, or fistulizing disease, not only located in the anastomosis, would suggest a diagnosis of Crohn. The distinction of de novo Crohn's disease from chronic antibiotic resistant pouchitis or technical complications related to surgery is however often difficult. Clinical symptoms, endoscopic features, and radiographic findings may all look similar in suspected de novo Crohn of the pouch and other pouch morbidities.

Complications to pouch surgery can result in a Crohn-like clinical picture with fistulas, abscesses or strictures. The time to pouch-related complications from ileostomy takedown or the anatomic disease location may provide clues for an accurate diagnosis. A short duration from stoma closure to onset of a fistula probably represents a leak and makes the diagnosis of Crohn unlikely, as does a fistula originating from the anastomosis or suture line. On the other hand, a long duration after surgery (more than 12 months) to onset of symptoms after an interval without postoperative local complications and with normal pouch function suggests de novo Crohn's disease. Crohn's disease is also suspected if a fistula fails to respond to repeated surgical repairs. The anatomic location of stricturing (e.g. proximal ileum versus the pouch anastomosis) can also be helpful making the diagnosis, because anastomotic stricturing is likely related to surgery, whereas proximal small-bowel stricturing could indicate Crohn. Segmental disease distribution, and potential involvement of other parts of the gastrointestinal tract can also be useful in differential diagnosis. Involvement of more proximal parts of the gastrointestinal tract would strongly indicate Crohn.

Pre-pouch ileitis can have an appearance that closely resembles Crohn with erosions and ulcerations. It has been considered to predict Crohn's disease, but is now increasingly understood not to necessarily represent development of a de novo Crohn. It is rather a form of backwash ileitis associated with the pouchitis itself. It can extend up to 50 cm into the afferent limb and is also associated with stricturing. The cumulative incidence in retrospective studies has been about 6% of all patients with a pelvic pouch after colectomy for Ulcerative Colitis and 13% of those with pouchitis. In a European cohort, all patients with pre-pouch ileitis also had pouchitis.

Long-term follow up of a subgroup of this cohort showed that pre-pouch ileitis was associated with an increased risk of pouch failure, and that pre-pouch ileitis did not appear to be a strong predictor of reclassification to Crohn's disease.

The differential diagnostics is thus difficult and often empiric, with a sliding transition to a more and more probable diagnosis of Crohn. In a study from the US 80% of patients undergoing pouch excision for Crohn of the pouch did not have pathology consistent with Crohn at the time of pouch excision. Making an accurate diagnosis of Crohn of the pouch versus a postoperative complication is important for both decisions regarding medical management, and pouch excision versus reconstruction. Most patients diagnosed with Crohn's disease will no longer be considered for pouch reconstructive surgery.

To increase the diagnostic accuracy for Crohn a thorough assessment is necessary of both the pouch and the rest of the gastrointestinal tract including endoscopy, histology, and radiography, as well as tests (including cultures) to rule out infectious enteritis.

Endoscopy of the pouch and the prepouch ileum, including biopsies, is the first-line procedure to discriminate pouchitis from other mimicking disorders. Pouchitis usually shows a diffuse inflammation involving the whole pouch. Crohn's disease of the pouch and pouchitis often has similar mucosal features, and morphologic characteristics of ulcers in the pouch are generally not reliable for a distinction between the two conditions. As stated above inflammation of the pre-pouch ileum is in itself not diagnostic for Crohn. Strictures or fistulization in the pouch or pre-pouch ileum could indicate Crohn, but also be due to surgical complications.

If Crohn's disease is suspected examination for additional lesions can be helpful. The upper gastrointestinal tract is examined by endoscopy and the small bowel by computed tomography (CT), magnetic resonance imaging (MRI) or trans-abdominal ultrasonography (US), which all have high and similar accuracy to assess Crohn's of the small bowel. They can establish disease extent and inflammatory activity, differentiate between inflammatory or fibrotic components of a stricture, judge the functional effects of a stricture from prestenotic dilatation, and diagnose penetrating disease. In selected patients with suspicion of more proximal small bowel disease, despite normal radiological examinations, capsule endoscopy can give further information, as well as double ballon enteroscopy.

Histopathological examination can be useful to rule out differential diagnoses, but adds little to distinguish Crohn from antibiotic-refractory chronic pouchitis. Typical histological findings in Crohn's disease are transmural inflammation, focal crypt irregularity (colon) or irregular villous architecture (ileum), patchy distribution of chronic inflammation in untreated patients, and granulomas. However, mucosal biopsies are too superficial to allow assessment of transmural inflammation, and granuloma formation is a rare finding. Only 10–12% of patients with known Crohn of the pouch have granulomas on mucosal biopsy and only granulomas in the lamina propria, not associated with active crypt injury, should be considered as a corroborative feature of Crohn. Moreover, biopsies from a staple line may yield foreign-body granuloma that falsely indicates Crohn's disease.

Considering the diagnostic difficulties a multidisciplinary approach including gastroenterologist, colorectal surgeon, pathologist (with a focus on gastroenterology), and radiologist is ideal. The response to medical and surgical management can give additional clues and the diagnosis may have to be reevaluated with an open mind.

15.2 Pathogenesis

The clinical entity of de novo Crohn of the pouch is not clearly defined and the pathogenesis of the change from a Ulcerative Colitis phenotype preoperatively to a Crohn-like phenotype of the pouch is not well understood, although it is recognized that these changes between phenotypes occur. The etiology of IBD is unknown and the pathophysiology is far from completely understood. The current main hypothesis for the onset of IBD is that the mucosal integrity is broken and environmental factors trigger a dysregulated immune system to react to one or more luminal factors, in a genetically predisposed host.

Whether IBD is one, two or several diseases with different phenotypes is unknown. IBD includes complex and heterogeneous disease phenotypes which raises the question if the different IBD phenotypes could be explained by different etiologies or if it rather is one common etiology resulting in different IBD phenotypes depending on how the immune system tends to react to it? Different genetic (IBD risk loci) and environmental factors (e.g. smoking) would then contribute to the modulation of the immune response into these phenotypes.

Currently IBD is divided into two entities, Crohn's disease and Ulcerative Colitis, based on the two main phenotypes. They are separated by disease presentation (anatomical distribution in the gut, endoscopic and histopathological features, risk for fibro-stenotic complications, and response to treatment), and different environmental (e.g. smoking) and genetic (susceptibility loci specific for either entity) risk factors. It could be argued that these two entities are still too heterogeneous and should be further divided into more homogenous disease subentities to allow better understanding of pathophysiology, prognosis, and management.

On the other hand, IBD could also be seen as a heterogeneous and continuous disease spectrum with different inflammatory phenotypes. In 5–10% of patients with IBD the clinical, endoscopic and histological features overlap and the phenotype is not possible to classify as Ulcerative Colitis or Crohn's disease. This is even more pronounced in children. This condition is called IBD-unclassified. If the colitis is still not possible to classify after histopathological examination of the colectomy specimen the diagnosis is indeterminate colitis. Over the disease course the phenotype often become clearer making it possible to define the condition as Ulcerative Colitis or Crohn's disease. Furthermore, the phenotype of a patient diagnosed with Ulcerative Colitis may change over time into Crohn, or vice versa, in 5–10% of patients.

Parent-child, twin and sibling studies have provided evidence that genetic predisposition to IBD increases the risk of developing IBD, more so in Crohn's disease than in Ulcerative Colitis. The concordance for disease type is however far from complete, even in monozygotic twins. In a Norwegian study the disease concordance for parent–child pairs was 52% for Ulcerative Colitis and 88% for Crohn, and 70% for sib-sib pairs in both Ulcerative Colitis and Crohn. Genetic components are important factors involved in the disease pathogenesis, and the identification of risk loci in IBD has increased the understanding of possible pathophysiological mechanisms involved, but most of the risk loci are common in the population, with a modest increase in risk and a low penetrance, and therefore the disease variance explained by these IBD risk loci is low, 13.6% and 7.5% for Crohn and Ulcerative Colitis, respectively.

The contribution of environmental factors, mostly still unknown, thus seems to play the most important role in the development of IBD. This is further underlined by the fact that the incidence in the world is increasing over time, especially in countries assuming a western way of living or in population groups moving from geographic areas with low to high IBD incidence. Smoking has repeatedly been shown to influence the phenotypic disease expression in persons with heritability for IBD, with smokers tending to develop Crohn.

It is hypothesized that host–bacteria interactions trigger chronic bowel inflammation. Several studies have reported that IBD patients have a dysbiosis of the intestinal microbiota compared with that in healthy subjects, but it is yet not clear whether this is a cause or a result of the inflammatory process. Data on the association between use of antibiotics and risk of developing IBD have been conflicting, but in a recent study antibiotic use was associated with an increased risk of IBD onset, both for Ulcerative Colitis and Crohn. If dysbiosis in itself was a driver of inflammation in IBD it could be anticipated that treatments directed towards the microbiota would influence outcome. However, antibiotics and probiotics does not seem to have an evident role for induction of remission in active Ulcerative Colitis, and fecal microbiota transplantation has so far shown limited and conflicting results. Antibiotics and probiotics are not effective for active luminal Crohn, and the limited data available for fecal microbiota transplantation for Crohn have not been convincing.

The etiology of pouchitis is also unknown. The effect of short courses of antibiotics and probiotics for pouchitis, compared to the limited effect in Ulcerative Colitis and Crohn, suggests that the underlying cause of pouchitis is mainly attributable to microbial dysbiosis or bacterial overgrowth. Several studies describe bacterial dysbiosis in patients with pouchitis. The construction of a pouch results in an altered bowel environment, and fecal stasis may increase the risk for dysbiosis. Patients with familial adenomatous polyposis (FAP) undergo the same pouch procedure as patients with Ulcerative Colitis. The overall rate of postoperative complications is reported to be similar for FAP and Ulcerative Colitis. The risk of pouchitis in FAP patients is however much lower (approximately 5%), and with a milder course, although recent studies indicate that pouchitis in FAP patients would not be as infrequent as previously believed.

A reasonable explanation for this difference would be that an acquired dysregulated immune response in patients with IBD increases the risk of developing pouchitis. The ileal mucosa of the pouch, irrespective of original diagnosis, can change into a more colon-like phenotype with villous atrophy, crypt hyperplasia, and change from small intestinal type sialyated mucin to highly sulfated colorectal-type mucin. It has been suggested that this would be an adaptive response to fecal stasis and dysbiosis including sulfate-reducing bacteria, and that presentation of colon-specific antigens may activate the already triggered immune system in IBD-patients, but not so in patients with FAP. This could then be an explanation for the development into a chronic antibiotic resistant pouchitis, or even a Crohn's disease-like phenotype, in patients with IBD. There are differences in microbiota between IBD-patients with pouchitis and a normal pouch, and also compared to patients with FAP pouch with sulfate reducing bacteria in the majority of Ulcerative Colitis patients but none in FAP patients. The expression of sulphomucin is increased in the mucous gel layer of Ulcerative Colitis compared with FAP pouches. Differential mucin expression favours colonization of different organisms and sulphomucin expression is associated with sulphate-reducing bacteria and increased chronic inflammation. What is the chicken or the egg is however still unclear.

15.3 Risk of Recurrence of Crohn's Disease or Developing de Novo Crohn's Disease After Colectomy for IBD

The risk of recurrence of CD in the neoterminal ileum after colectomy for Crohn's colitis has been considered to be low as long as the patient has an ileostomy. The onset of inflammation in Crohn has been thought to be triggered by the fecal stream once an ileo-colonic anastomosis has been constructed with a clinical recurrence rate of about 50% after 10 years. Developing de novo Crohn in the small bowel in patients with ileostomy after colectomy for Ulcerative Colitis has been considered a rarity. Recent publications have somewhat challenged these views.

In a meta-analysis of 14 studies with a total of 1004 patients the risk of clinical recurrence of Crohn's disease after total colectomy with permanent ileostomy was reported to be 28%. After 5 and 10 years, the cumulative recurrence rate of clinical Crohn was 24% and 40%, respectively. Patients with ileal disease had a 3-fold increased risk of clinical recurrence. In six studies reporting the location of recurrence in 132 patients, 81% experienced ileal, and 14% extensive small bowel recurrence, whereas 3% had jejunal, and 2% upper gastrointestinal tract recurrence. For patients without history of ileal disease the clinical recurrence rate was 12% based on three studies.

In a retrospective study a single centre cohort of colectomized Ulcerative Colitis patients with either pelvic pouch or permanent ileostomy, was followed for a mean of 20 years. After an average of 5 years 32 of 128 Ulcerative Colitis patients (25%) had developed de novo Crohn's Disease in the small bowel. There was no significant difference in risk of de novo Crohn between patients with a pelvic pouch or permanent ileostomy.

In another retrospective study 123 patients with permanent ileostomy after colectomy for Ulcerative Colitis were followed over a median of 5 years. Patients with secondary ileostomy after failing a pouch (n = 66) had a significantly higher risk of de novo Crohn of the small bowel compared with the 57 patients having primary ileostomy (46% vs. 9%, p < 0.001). Risk factors for de novo Crohn of the small bowel were failure of pouch, family history of IBD and postoperative history of weight loss. Of those failing their pelvic pouch 9% already had de novo Crohn of the pouch.

Patients with Crohn's Disease who undergo pouch surgery have a clearly increased risk of recurrence of Crohn and higher incidence of pouch failure, when compared with those who have Ulcerative Colitis or indeterminate colitis. A preoperative diagnosis of Crohn's disease is therefore generally considered a contraindication to pouch surgery because of the increased risk of recurrence of complicated Crohn resulting in pouch dysfunction, a higher rate of pouch excision, and the potential for short-bowel syndrome.

The reported rates of de novo Crohn after pelvic pouch and proctocolectomy for Ulcerative Colitis vary between 3% and 25%. The wide range in prevalence reflects the retrospective design of these studies, difficulty to differentiate Crohn from surgical complications, and lack of uniform diagnostic criteria to define de novo Crohn, but also differences in clinical settings, referral bias and intensity and duration of follow-up between the studies.

De novo Crohn's disease of the pouch is associated with a high risk for pouch removal. Pouch failure is reported in about 50 per cent of patients, but with considerable variation depending on the study related factors mentioned above, the treatment strategies used to prevent failure, and the local indications for pouch resection. The risk for de novo Crohn or pouch failure does not seem to differ between Ulcerative Colitis, IBD-U and indeterminate colitis, even though results are not consistent. Reported risk factors for developing de novo Crohn's disease include a family history of Crohn, being an active smoker and seropositive anti-Saccharomyces cerevisiae IgA (ASCA). All these factors are associated with Crohn's disease and could mean that the patient already had a tendency for developing a Crohn-like phenotype.

15.4 Treatment

There is very limited data on the medical management of de novo Crohn of pouches and the study quality is often poor. It is mainly restricted to retrospective, open, uncontrolled case series, with in-homogenous treatment strategies, in small cohorts of patients with pelvic pouches. No randomized controlled trials have been performed for de novo Crohn neither in pelvic pouches, nor continent ileostomies. The knowledge we can use in the management of de novo Crohn of the continent ileostomy therefore is mainly taken from management of IBD in general and Crohn's disease in particular. Then we must keep in mind that the reason most of these patients got operated and had a pouch was because they were treatment refractory. Little is known about how this may influence the treatment outcome of their new inflammatory state.

Immediate postoperative and long-term complications are common with continent ileostomy and leads to a high reoperation rate. Still the removal rate is low, which underlines that many patients highly appreciate their continent ileostomy for preserving fecal continence and improving the body image compared to common ileostomy. It also shows how complex and challenging the clinical decisions can be for both patient and the medico-surgical team to value risks and benefits to achieve the best possible long-term health for the patient. A successful management is thus facilitated by cooperation in a multidisciplinary team with gastroenterologists and colorectal surgeons, closely involving the patient in therapeutic decisions with a person centered approach.

The ultimate goal is the best possible health for the patient. There is a good chance of achieving a satisfactory pouch function and preserved quality of life with a combination of medical, nutritional, endoscopic, and surgical approaches, but prolonged hopeless attempts to restore the pouch function must be avoided. A conventional ileostomy could objectively be a better alternative to preserving a poorly functioning pouch, need of repeated surgical revisions with risk of perioperative complications and/or costly and potentially harmful immunosuppressive drugs.

As previously mentioned there is a high risk of misdiagnosing a patient with a Crohn-like phenotype and management is therefore often challenging. This may have considerable consequences. Patients with Crohn's disease being treated as having surgery-associated complications have a high risk of poor postoperative outcome, when they would have had a fair chance to respond to anti-inflammatory drugs. Patients with surgical complications being mislabeled as Crohn will on the other hand probably respond poorly to anti-inflammatory drugs and risk exclusion from pouch reconstructive surgery, although they may have had good long-term results after a salvage operation. The diagnostic decision thus influences the choice of reconstructive surgery or pharmacological treatment. In patients with a high probability of Crohn a new attempt with reconstruction should be avoided. However, if the Crohn diagnosis is uncertain with a fair probability that the disorder is due to surgical complications after careful evaluation, an attempt for reconstruction can be successful. In comparison with those patients undergoing a primary pelvic pouch, functional results after pouch redo were similar.

The diagnostic workup is thus vital to achieve the right understanding of the problem including the probability that it actually is de novo Crohn versus surgical complications. The presence of active inflammation due to Crohn's disease should be confirmed with endoscopy or inflammatory markers before starting or changing medical therapy. Alternative explanations for symptoms such as enteric infection, abscess, bacterial overgrowth, and dysmotility should be considered. Distribution of disease is re-evaluated if the clinical presentation over time changes or if it will affect medical or surgical management.

If the diagnosis is still not conclusive, the management has to be pragmatic. Response to different medical or surgical treatments with tight follow up and monitoring can be attempted. For example, the outcome of attempts with surgical repairs or an anti-TNF may help separate fistulizing Crohn's disease from surgically induced leaks or fistulae.

The management plan for a patient with Crohn's disease has to consider the severity, extent, and location of disease, intestinal complications or extra-intestinal manifestations, and previous treatment response. The goal is to induce and maintain steroid free clinical remission and if possible sustained inflammatory control to prevent relapses and future complications. The balance between the potential risks with a strategy and the chance of long-term success is important to consider. Treat to target, tight control and a preset time point for final evaluation when treatment is expected to have had its chance to work are important principles. The strategy to maintain remission should be considered early on and be part of management already during induction of remission. The risk of a poor disease course may be predicted from known clinical factors and should be considered when determining the therapeutic strategy.

The current clinical practice of medical management of IBD, including de novo Crohn in patients with a pouch, is primarily based on a rapid 'step up' approach with a hierarchic order of therapeutic strategies based on effectiveness, side effects and costs, where failure of one strategy to reach the goal within the expected time frame leads to the next until a strategy is successful. However, for patients with severe, extensive or complicated disease indicating a poor prognosis early combination therapy with biologics and immuno-modulators should be considered to achieve control of the disease as quickly as possible. Several studies have shown that anti-TNF therapy is more effective when initiated early in the disease course. If this is applicable also to de novo Crohn of the pouch we do not know, but it is still a reasonable strategy in severe cases. If and when the inflammation is under full control one may consider to slowly de-escalate therapy under tight monitoring with endoscopy, radiological imaging or guiding biomarkers as CRP and fecal calprotectin to assure that inflammatory control is maintained.

For clinical management and prognosis of Crohn's disease of the pouch it can be helpful to divide the disease behavior into inflammatory, fibro-stenotic, or fistulizing phenotype, modified from the Montreal classification. The hierarchical nature of the Montreal classification based on the worst phenotype at any time during the disease course may not always be clinically relevant. Fibro-stenotic and fistulizing disease can be present simultaneously, either can dominate at different time points during the disease course, and penetrating complications tends to be related to stricturing and active intestinal inflammation. Still it is a clinically relevant way to structure the current disease challenges and come up with a management strategy to handle them with combined medical and surgical therapies.

15.4.1 Inflammatory Phenotype

Antibiotics, including ciprofloxacin, metronidazole and rifaximin, are effective for pouchitis in the majority of patients. Therefore, in patients with pouchitis, including those with backwash ileitis, antibiotics (e.g. ciprofloxacin 1000 mg daily and metronidazole 1000 mg daily, or rifaximin 2000 mg daily) for at least 4 weeks should be tried before considering anti-inflammatory medication. In antibiotic-dependent pouchitis low-dose ciprofloxacin, or rifaximin can be given as maintenance therapy. An alternative for patients in remission could be maintenance treatment with the probiotic VSL#3. In antibiotic resistant chronic pouchitis the inflammation may respond to anti-inflammatory drugs used for IBD and the pharmacological strategies used for IBD could be applied although data about the effectiveness of 5-ASA, immune-modulators, or biologics in antibiotic refractory pouchitis or Crohn-like pouchitis are of poor quality or non-existing. Depending on the extent of the disease different applications can be used. If the inflammation is limited to the pouch topical treatments may be effective. If the inflammation involves the pre-pouch ileum or the more proximal gastrointestinal tract oral treatment is added. Therapy resistant cases or cases with a Crohn-like phenotype may respond to anti-TNF or vedolizumab, and if not, surgical reconstruction or excision may be required.

15.4.1.1 Induction Therapy with Steroids

The choice of steroid and application depends on the severity and location of Crohn's disease. For mild-moderate inflammation budesonide can be given as enema or foam for local treatment of the ileal pouch, but if both the pre-pouch ileum and the ileal pouch is involved oral budesonide 9 mg daily can be added for 8 weeks. The effect of budesonide is mainly local in the gut and, due to high first pass metabolism in the liver, it has lower systemic side effects than prednisolone. Budesonide is however less effective than prednisolone. In more severe or extended inflammatory Crohn's disease oral prednisolon given as a course of initially 30–40 mg tapered with 5 mg per week and/or with local steroids (foam or enema) is more effective for induction of remission. Treatment with systemic steroids should be restricted since they may result in well-known, potentially severe, side effects, and increase the susceptibility to serious infections, especially in combination with other immune-suppressive agents.

Steroids are effective at inducing short term remission, but are ineffective at maintaining remission. In the short term patients treated with steroids can turn out to be steroid refractory or intolerant, become steroid dependent, or enter remission. A prednisolone tapering course starting at doses of 40–60 mg will induce short term complete or partial clinical remission in up to about 80% of patients with active CD (144–148). The remainder of patients is termed steroid refractory. About 30% will end up steroid dependent, i.e. be unable to withdraw steroids without relapsing during tapering or within 3 months of stopping steroids. At 1 year after stopping steroids only about 40% will have prolonged steroid free clinical remission without surgery. The long-term strategy should therefore be planned early on.

15.4.1.2 Remission

If the disease is mild and clinical and endoscopic remission is achieved on steroids, one may not need to provide maintenance treatment, but instead await the course of the disease. In case of prognostic unfavorable disease, or rapid or frequent relapses immune-modulators and/or biologics are introduced as maintenance therapy early on. Patients in remission should be monitored on a regular basis with CRP and fecal calprotectin to assess disease activity and optimize treatment if needed.

15.4.1.3 Steroid Refractory Disease

Early introduction of anti-TNF therapy is needed in steroid-refractory or steroid intolerant patients. Anti-TNFs are effective in Crohn's disease and available real world data (RWD) mainly for infliximab, but to some extent also adalimumab, has shown good effect in antibiotic refractory or Crohn-like pouchitis. Combination therapy with anti-TNF and thiopurines in Crohn patients naïve to both drugs is more effective than anti-TNF monotherapy in achieving corticosteroid-free clinical remission and complete mucosal healing. The thiopurines, mercaptopurine and its prodrug azathioprine, are effective for inducing and maintaining remission in Crohn's disease. However, thiopurines have slow onset and are therefore not suitable for induction of remission as monotherapy, but they reduce the risk of anti-drug antibody formation and can also contribute with an additive effect after 3–6 months (median at 4.5 months). After 6–12 months with combo therapy in patients previously naïve to both anti-TNF and azathioprine one may consider to stop anti-TNF and continue azathioprine as mono maintenance therapy. To consider this patient's should have complete inflammatory control. It is recommended to monitor tightly for recurrence of inflammation. In case this strategy does not succeed despite adequate thiopurine dosage, anti-TNF is reintroduced.

The dosing of thiopurines is initially weight based with azathioprine 1.5–2.5 mg/kg and mercaptopurine 1.0–1.5 mg/kg. The metabolism of thiopurines is however complicated and individual. Drug discontinuation occurs in up to 50% of cases due to side effects or failure of therapy. Pre-treatment testing of TPMT and therapeutic drug monitoring (TDM) is therefore recommended to adjust dosing to better achieve effect and handle adverse events.

Dosing to achieve tioguanin nucleotides between 250 and 450 pmol/8×10^8 RBC makes clinical efficacy more likely and avoids side effects of unnecessary high tioguanin nucleotides levels. Approximately 14% have skewed metabolism with low tioguanin nucleotides levels and high methylated metabolites which may lead to lower effect and more side effects and can be effectively handled with co-administration with allopurinol and azathioprine/mercaptopurine reduced to 25–33% of the monotherapy dose. Switch from azathioprine to mercaptopurine may be a successful strategy in approximately 50% of patients with more general side effects, but not in cases with idiosyncratic reactions such as pancreatitis.

Methotrexate is an alternative, mainly in patients intolerant of thiopurines. Methotrexate has a slow onset over 2–3 months. For induction methotrexate 25 mg s.c. or i.m. is given once weekly for 4 months. Supplementation with folic acid 5–10 mg is recommended 1–2 days following methotrexate to reduce side effects. If induction treatment is successful the dosage is lowered to a maintenance dosage of 15 mg weekly after 4 months. In Crohn's disease methotrexate is usually given as s.c. or i.m. injections, since oral dosing has highly variable bioavailability and comparative effectiveness studies of oral and subcutaneous methotrexate are lacking.

Thiopurines can prevent and reverse immunogenicity against biologics. In patients with thiopurine failure despite adequate tioguanin nucleotides levels one may therefore consider to use it merely to prevent immunogenicity and loss of response. For this indication it appears possible to reduce the azathioprine/mercaptopurine dose to a dosage equivalent to a tioguanin nucleotides level above 125 pmol/8 × 10^8 red blood cells. In patients with loss-of-response to biological therapy due to anti-drug antibody formation, addition of an immune-modulator can reverse the immunogenicity, leading to a regained response. In patients intolerant to thiopurines, methotrexate can be an alternative to prevent immunogenicity. Since combination therapy with anti-TNFs and thiopurines may increase the risk for malignancies and infections one has to individualize the choice of treatment. The need of preventing immunogenicity with combination therapy is much higher with the chimeric monoclonal antibody infliximab compared to the humanized monoclonal antibodies, e.g. adalimumab, vedolizumab and ustekinumab. In patients considered for anti-TNF monotherapy adalimumab may therefore be preferred.

15.4.1.4   Steroid Dependent Disease

Patients responding to high steroid doses, but who relapses during tapering or shortly after stopping steroids (<3 months) are considered to be steroid dependent. For steroid dependent patients immunomodulators and/or biologics are usually appropriate to achieve steroid free remission. If the long-term maintenance treatment is planned to be thiopurines the patient is given lowest possible steroid dose to keep the disease under control until thiopurines has become efficacious after 3–6 months. Then steroids are tapered and stopped. If the patient is steroid dependent on a high dose (>20 mg prednisolone) anti-TNF treatment is considered to enable a faster tapering of steroids to minimize side effects. In patients with thiopurine failure despite dose optimization to a tioguanin nucleotides level between 250 and 450, anti-TNF is first line biologic. In case of failure to immunomodulators and anti-TNF other biologic agents approved for CD, such as the anti-$\alpha4\beta7$-integrin vedolizumab or the anti-IL12/23 p40 antibody ustekinumab, may be considered.

In primary non-responders to induction or loss of response (relapse after initially having achieved remission at 3 months) on anti-TNF, dose optimization is considered, usually after checking drug serum levels. If drug serum levels are low, without anti-drug antibody formation, increased dosage is recommended. In case of low serum levels and presence of anti-drug antibody the best option would be to switch within class. If there is no response despite adequate serum levels a swap to another class of biologics is considered. At present the alternatives for Crohn's disease are vedolizumab or ustekinumab.

In patients with failure to immunomudulators (thiopurines and methothrexate) and biologics (anti-TNF, vedolizumab, and ustekinumab), despite therapeutic drug monitoring with optimized dosing, excision of the pouch has to be considered. Surgery is a reasonable alternative for patients with disease refractory to medical treatment and should be discussed as an alternative at every step up of the therapy. The therapeutic strategy for an individual should be a joint decision between the patient, gastroenterologist and colorectal surgeon.

15.4.2 Fibro-Stenotic Crohn's Disease

For fibro-stenotic Crohn, a combined medical, endoscopic and surgical management is often needed. Differentiation between inflammatory and fibro-stenotic strictures is crucial to the choice of therapy. If the inflammatory component is dominating steroids are often successful to swell off the inflammatory edema that obstructs the bowel lumen. In patients responding to steroids immuno-modulators and/or anti-TNF are usually given as maintenance therapy with the aim of controlling the inflammation and trying to delay the fibro-stenotic process that may eventually lead to stricturing and the need of endoscopic or surgical intervention, even though data is scarce. If steroids are un-effective the fibro-stenotic component is probably already too large for success with anti-inflammatory drugs. If a symptomatic stricture is short (<4 cm) endoscopic balloon dilation is the preferred technique as a conservative strategy in combination with medical management to avoid or postpone the need for surgical intervention. Surgical options include strictureplasty or resection. Conventional strictureplasty is advised when the length of the stricture is <10 cm, as a safe and potentially bowel-sparing strategy for small bowel Crohn, compared to resection. For patients with pouch strictures, periodic endoscopic therapy or surgical strictureplasty may help reduce the risk for pouch-diverting surgery.

15.4.3 Fistulizing Crohn's Disease

In patients with an ileal pouch, the development of fistulas results in severe morbidity with a significant risk of reservoir loss. The management of fistulizing Crohn of a continent pouch can be difficult and usually requires a combined medical and surgical approach. Data is scarce and there are no RCTs on the effect of medical treatment for non-perianal fistulizing Crohn other than the subgroups of several trials. There are only retrospective real world data investigating the role of anti-TNF therapy in patients with antibiotic refractory pouchitis or Crohn-like fistulizing or stricturing disease. Management recommendations therefore mainly have to be applied from the more common and better studied perianal fistulization.

Fistulizing Crohn's disease in patients with a continent pouch comprises fistulae communicating between the pouch or pre-pouch intestine and other parts of the intestine, other organs or the abdominal wall. The origin of the fistula has to be located and the fistula anatomy and which organs it affects have to be determined. Active luminal inflammation or strictures has to be assessed, including the intestine where the fistula originates. Presence of local sepsis (abscess) has to be evaluated with MRI, CT or US. A meta-analysis found thiopurines to be effective for perianal fistulization and thiopurines appear effective both for fistula closing and closure maintenance, but there is no data for fistulizing Crohn's disease of the pouch. The effect of infliximab or adalimumab on perianal fistula closure was evaluated in placebo controlled RCTs, and about one third had complete fistula closure at week 54 with infliximab and at week 56 with adalimumab.

The experience of infliximab and adalimumab in pouch patients only comes from retrospective real world data in patients with chronic pouchitis or Crohn's disease of the pouch. Based on these data a combination of thiopurines and anti-TNF is recommended for fistulizing Crohn's disease of the pouch, but the experience is that internal fistulas respond less well to anti-TNF treatment compared to perianal fistulas and often require surgery. If an abscess is present it has to be drained before start of anti-inflammatory treatment. Antibiotics improve symptoms in perianal fistula and combination of anti-TNF and ciprofloxacin had better effect on perianal fistula closure than anti-TNF monotherapy in a 12 week trial. Entero-enteric fistulas associated with a stricture need surgical management. Low output enterocutaneous fistulae can be treated with immune-modulators and anti-TNF, whereas high output fistulae and fistulae complicated with abscess or stricture needs surgery.

Bibliography

1. Simchuk EJ, Thirlby RC. Risk factors and true incidence of pouchitis in patients after ileal pouch-anal anastomoses. World J Surg. 2000;24:851–6.
2. Penna C, Dozois R, Tremaine W, et al. Pouchitis after ileal pouch-anal anastomosis for ulcerative colitis occurs with increased frequency in patients with associated primary sclerosing cholangitis. Gut. 1996;38:234–9.
3. Romanos J, Samarasekera DN, Stebbing JF, et al. Outcome of 200 restorative proctocolectomy operations: the John Radcliffe hospital experience. Br J Surg. 1997;84:814–8.
4. Svaninger G, Nordgren S, Oresland T, et al. Incidence and characteristics of pouchitis in the Kock continent ileostomy and the pelvic pouch. Scand J Gastroenterol. 1993;28:695–700.
5. Hahnloser D, Pemberton JH, Wolff BG, et al. Results at up to 20 years after ileal pouch-anal anastomosis for chronic ulcerative colitis. Br J Surg. 2007;94:333–40.
6. Banasiewicz T, Marciniak R, Kaczmarek E, et al. The prognosis of clinical course and the analysis of the frequency of the inflammation and dysplasia in the intestinal J-pouch at the patients after restorative proctocolectomy due to FAP. Int Colorectal Dis. 2011;26:1197–203.
7. Meagher AP, Farouk R, Dozois RR, et al. J-ileal pouch anal anastomosis for chronic ulcerative colitis: complications and long-term outcome in 1310 patients. Br J Surg. 1998;85:800–3.
8. Lovegrove RE, Tilney HS, Heriot AG, et al. A comparison of adverse events and functional outcomes after restorative protocolectomy for familial adenoma-Tous polyposis and ulcerative colitis. Dis Colon Rectum. 2006;49:1293–306.
9. Zaghiyan K, Kamiński JP, Barmparas G, Fleshner P. De novo Crohn's disease after ileal pouch anal anastomosis for ulcerative colitis and inflammatory bowel disease unclassified: long-term follow-up of a prospective inflammatory bowel disease registry. Am Surg. 2016;82:977–81.
10. Shen B. Crohn's disease of the ileal pouch: reality, diagnosis, and management. Inflamm Bowel Dis. 2009;15:284–94.

11. Lennard-Jones JE, Shivananda S. Clinical uniformity of inflammatory bowel disease a presentation and during the first year of disease in the north and south of Europe. EC-IBD study group. Eur J Gastroenterol Hepatol. 1997;9:353–9.
12. Shen B, Fazio VW, Remzi FH, et al. Risk factors for clinical phenotypes of Crohn's disease of the pouch. Am J Gastroenterol. 2006;101:2760–8.
13. Wolf JM, Achkar J-P, Lashner BA, et al. Afferent limb ulcers predict Crohn's disease in patients with ileal pouch-anal anastomosis. Gastroenterology. 2004;126:1686–91.
14. Shen B, Fazio VW, Remzi FH, et al. Comprehensive evaluation of inflammatory and noninflammatory sequelae of ileal pouchanal anastomoses. Am J Gastroenterol. 2005;100:93–101.
15. Deutsch AA, McLeod RS, Cullen J, Cohen Z. Results of the pelvic-pouch procedure in patients with Crohn's disease. Dis Colon Rectum. 1991;34:475–7.
16. Grobler SP, Hosie KB, Keighley MR. Randomized trial of loop ileostomy in restorative proctocolectomy. Br J Surg. 1992;79:903–6.
17. Hyman NH, Fazio VW, Tuckson WB, Lavery IC. Consequences of ileal pouch-anal anastomosis for Crohn's colitis. Dis Colon Rectum. 1991;34:653–7.
18. Shen B, Fazio VW, Remzi FH, et al. Clinical features and quality of life in patients with different phenotypes of Crohn's disease of the ileal pouch. Dis Colon Rectum. 2007;50:1450–9.
19. Stein RB, Lichtenstein GR. Complications after ileal pouch-anal anastomosis. Semin Gastrointest Dis. 2000;11:2–9.
20. Shen B, Fazio VW, Remzi FH, Lashner BA. Clinical approach to diseases of ileal pouch-anal anastomosis. Am J Gastroenterol. 2005;100:2796–807.
21. Lightner AL, Fletcher JG, Pemberton JH, et al. Crohn's disease of the pouch: a true diagnosis or an oversubscribed diagnosis of exclusion? Dis Colon Rectum. 2017;60:1201–8.
22. Tekkis PP, Fazio VW, Remzi F, et al. Risk factors associated with ileal pouch-related fistula following restorative proctocolectomy. Br J Surg. 2005;92:1270–6.
23. Ferrante M, D'Haens G, Dewit O, et al. Efficacy of infliximab in refractory pouchitis and Crohn's disease-related complications of the pouch: a Belgian case series. Inflamm Bowel Dis. 2010;16:243–9.
24. Bell AJ, Price AB, Forbes A, et al. Pre-pouch ileitis: a disease of the ileum in ulcerative colitis after restorative proctocolectomy. Color Dis. 2006;8:402–10.
25. McLaughlin SD, Clark SK, Bell AJ, et al. Incidence and short-term implications of prepouch ileitis following restorative proctocolectomy with ileal pouch-anal anastomosis for ulcerative colitis. Dis Colon Rectum. 2009;52:879–83.
26. Samaan MA, de Jong D, Sahami S, et al. Incidence and severity of prepouch ileitis: a distinct disease entity or a manifestation of refractory pouchitis? Inflamm Bowel Dis. 2016;22:662–8.
27. Segal JP, McLaughlin SD, Faiz OD, Clark SK, Hart AL. Incidence and long-term implications of prepouch ileitis: an observational study. Dis Colon Rectum. 2018;23 [Epub ahead of print].
28. Fraquelli M, Colli A, Casazza G, et al. Role of US in detection of Crohn disease: meta-analysis. Radiology. 2005;236:95–101.
29. Koh DM, Miao Y, Chinn RJ, et al. MR imaging evaluation of the activity of Crohn's disease. Am J Roentgenol. 2001;177:1325–32.
30. Horsthuis K, Bipat S, Bennink RJ, et al. Inflammatory bowel disease diagnosed with US, MR, scintigraphy, and CT: meta-analysis of prospective studies. Radiology. 2008;247:64–79.
31. Panes J, Bouzas R, Chaparro M, et al. Systematic review: the use of ultrasonography, computed tomography and magnetic resonance imaging for the diagnosis, assessment of activity and abdominal complications of Crohn's disease. Aliment Pharmacol Ther. 2011;34:125–45.
32. Qiu Y, Mao R, Chen BL, et al. Systematic review with meta-analysis: magnetic resonance enterography vs. computed tomography enterography for evaluating disease activity in small bowel Crohn's disease. Aliment Pharmacol Ther. 2014;40:134–46.
33. Wold PB, Fletcher JG, Johnson CD, et al. Assessment of small bowel Crohn disease: noninvasive peroral CT enterography compared with other imaging methods and endoscopy-- feasibility study. Radiology. 2003;229:275–81.

34. Takenaka K, Ohtsuka K, Kitazume Y, Matsuoka K, Fujii T, Nagahori M, Kimura M, Fujioka T, Araki A, Watanabe M. Magnetic resonance evaluation for small bowel strictures in Crohn's disease: comparison with balloon enteroscopy. J Gastroenterol. 2017;52:879–88.
35. Rispo A, Imperatore N, Testa A, et al. Bowel damage in Crohn's disease: direct comparison of ultrasonography-based and magnetic resonance-based Lemann index. Inflamm Bowel Dis. 2017;23:143–51.
36. Tillack C, Seiderer J, Brand S, et al. Correlation of magnetic resonance enteroclysis (MRE) and wireless capsule endoscopy (CE) in the diagnosis of small bowel lesions in Crohn's disease. Inflamm Bowel Dis. 2008;14:1219–28.
37. Geboes K, Colombel JF, Greenstein A, et al. Pathology task force of the International Organization of Inflammatory Bowel Diseases. Indeterminate colitis: a review of the concept--what's in a name? Inflamm Bowel Dis. 2008;14:850–7.
38. Bernades P, Hecketsweiler P, Benozio M, et al. Proposal of a system of criteria for the diagnosis of cryptogenetic inflammatory enterocolitis (Crohn's disease and hemorrhagic rectocolitis). A cooperative study by the cryptogenic enterocolitis study group. Gastroenterol Clin Biol. 1978;2:1047–54.
39. Li Y, Wu B, Shen B. Diagnosis and differential diagnosis of Crohn's disease of the ileal pouch. Curr Gastroenterol Rep. 2012;14:406–13.
40. Garrett KA, Remzi FH, Kirat HT, et al. Outcome of salvage surgery for ileal pouches referred with a diagnosis of Crohn's disease. Dis Colon Rectum. 2009;52:1967–74.
41. Zundler S, Neurath MF. Immunopathogenesis of inflammatory bowel diseases: functional role of T cells and T cell homing. Clin Exp Rheumatol. 2015;33(4 Suppl 92):S19–28.
42. Sachar DB, Walfish A. Inflammatory bowel disease: one or two diseases? Curr Gastroenterol Rep. 2013;15:298.
43. Louis E, Van Kemseke C, Reenaers C. Necessity of phenotypic classification of inflammatory bowel disease. Best Pract Res Clin Gastroenterol. 2011;(25 Suppl 1):S2–7.
44. Yu YR, Rodriguez JR. Clinical presentation of Crohn's, ulcerative colitis, and indeterminate colitis: symptoms, extraintestinal manifestations, and disease phenotypes. Semin Pediatr Surg. 2017;26:349–55.
45. Ellinghaus D, Bethune J, Petersen BS, et al. The genetics of Crohn's disease and ulcerative colitis—status quo and beyond. Scand J Gastroenterol. 2015;50:13–23.
46. Bengtson MB, Solberg C, Aamodt G, et al. Clustering in time of familial IBD separates ulcerative colitis from Crohn's disease. Inflamm Bowel Dis. 2009;15:1867–74.
47. Molodecky NA, Soon IS, Rabi DM, et al. Increasing incidence and prevalence of the inflammatory bowel diseases with time, based on systematic review. Gastroenterology. 2012;142:46–54.
48. Kaplan GG, Ng SC. Understanding and preventing the global increase of inflammatory bowel disease. Gastroenterology. 2017;152:313–21.
49. Bridger S, Lee JC, Bjarnason I, et al. In siblings with similar genetic susceptibility for inflammatory bowel disease, smokers tend to develop Crohn's disease and non-smokers develop ulcerative colitis. Gut. 2002;51:21–5.
50. Nishida A, Inoue R, Inatomi O, et al. Gut microbiota in the pathogenesis of inflammatory bowel disease. Clin J Gastroenterol. 2018;11:1–10.
51. Theochari NA, Stefanopoulos A, Mylonas KS, Economopoulos KP. Antibiotics exposure and risk of inflammatory bowel disease: a systematic review. Scand J Gastroenterol. 2018;53:1–7.
52. Aniwan S, Tremaine WJ, Raffals LE, et al. Antibiotic use and new-onset inflammatory bowel disease in Olmsted county, Minnesota: a population-based case-control study. J Crohns Colitis. 2018;12:137–44.
53. Khan KJ, Ullman TA, Ford AC, et al. Antibiotic therapy in inflammatory bowel disease: a systematic review and meta-analysis. Am J Gastroenterol. 2011;106:661–73.
54. Orel R, Kamhi TT. Intestinal microbiota, probiotics and prebiotics in inflammatory bowel disease. World J Gastroenterol. 2014;20:11505–24.

55. Gomollón F, Dignass A, Annese V, et al. ECCO. 3rd European evidence-based consensus on the diagnosis and Management of Crohn's disease 2016: part 1: diagnosis and medical management. J Crohns Colitis. 2017;11:3–25.
56. Lohmuller JL, Pemberton JH, Dozois RR, et al. Pouchitis and extraintestinal manifestations of inflammatory bowel disease after ileal pouch-anal anastomosis. Ann Surg. 1990;211:622–7. discussion 7–9
57. Coffey JC, Rowan F, Burke J, et al. Pathogenesis of and unifying hypothesis for idiopathic pouchitis. Am J Gastroenterol. 2009;104:1013–23.
58. Wu H, Shen B. Pouchitis and pouch dysfunction. Med Clin North Am. 2010;94:75–92.
59. Cheifetz A, Itzkowitz S. The diagnosis and treatment of pouchitis in inflammatory bowel disease. J Clin Gastroenterol. 2004;38:S44–50.
60. Gionchetti P, Rizzello F, Venturi A, et al. Antibiotic combination therapy in patients with chronic, treatment-resistant pouchitis. Aliment Pharmacol Ther. 1999;13:713–8.
61. Shen B, Fazio VW, Remzi FH, et al. Combined ciprofloxacin and tinidazole therapy in the treatment of chronic refractory pouchitis. Dis Colon Rectum. 2007;50:498–508.
62. Isaacs KL, Sandler RS, Abreu M, et al. Rifaximin for the treatment of active pouchitis: a randomized, double-blind, placebo-controlled pilot study. Inflamm Bowel Dis. 2007;13:1250–5.
63. Madden MV, McIntyre AS, Nicholls RJ. Double-blind crossover trial of metronidazole versus placebo in chronic unremitting pouchitis. Dig Dis Sci. 1994;39:1193–6.
64. Mimura T, Rizzello F, Helwig U, et al. Four-week open-label trial of metronidazole and ciprofloxacin for the treatment of recurrent or refractory pouchitis. Aliment Pharmacol Ther. 2002;16:909–17.
65. Shen B, Achkar JP, Lashner BA, et al. A randomized clinical trial of ciprofloxacin and metronidazole to treat acute pouchitis. Inflamm Bowel Dis. 2001;7:301–5.
66. Holubar SD, Cima RR, Sandborn WJ, Pardi DS. Treatment and prevention of pouchitis after ileal pouch-anal anastomosis for chronic ulcerative colitis. Cochrane Database Syst Rev. 2010;6:CD001176.
67. Gionchetti P, Amadini C, Rizzello F, et al. Probiotics for the treatment of postoperative complications following intestinal surgery. Best Pract Res Clin Gastroenterol. 2003;17:821–31.
68. Gionchetti P, Rizzello F, Helwig U, et al. Prophylaxis of pouchitis onset with probiotic therapy: a double-blind, placebo-controlled trial. Gastroenterology. 2003;124:1202–9.
69. Shen B, Brzezinski A, Fazio VW, et al. Maintenance therapy with a probiotic in antibiotic-dependent pouchitis: experience in clinical practice. Aliment Pharmacol Ther. 2005;22:721–8.
70. Gionchetti P, Rizzello F, Morselli C, et al. High-dose probiotics for the treatment of active pouchitis. Dis Colon Rectum. 2007;50:2075–82.
71. Gionchetti P, Rizzello F, Venturi A, et al. Oral bacteriotherapy as maintenance treatment in patients with chronic pouchitis: a double-blind, placebo-controlled trial. Gastroenterology. 2000;119:305–9.
72. Mimura T, Rizzello F, Helwig U, et al. Once daily high dose probiotic therapy (VSL#3) for maintaining remission in recurrent or refractory pouchitis. Gut. 2004;53:108–14.
73. Lim M, Adams JD, Wilcox M, et al. An assessment of bacterial dysbiosis in pouchitis using terminal restriction fragment length polymorphisms of 16S ribosomal DNA from pouch effluent microbiota. Dis Colon Rectum. 2009;52:1492–500.
74. Sokol H, Lay C, Seksik P, et al. Analysis of bacterial bowel communities of IBD patients: what has it revealed? Inflamm Bowel Dis. 2008;14:858–67.
75. Komanduri S, Gillevet PM, Sikaroodi M, et al. Dysbiosis in Pouchitis: evidence of unique microfloral patterns in pouch inflammation. Clin Gastroenterol Hepatol. 2007;5:352–60.
76. McLaughlin SD, Clark SK, Tekkis PP, et al. The bacterial pathogenesis and treatment of pouchitis. Therap Adv Gastroenterol. 2010;3:335–48.
77. Quinn KP, Lightner AL, Pendegraft RS, et al. Pouchitis is a common complication in patients with familial adenomatous polyposis following ileal pouch-anal anastomosis. Clin Gastroenterol Hepatol. 2016;14:1296–301.

78. Salemans JM, Nagengast FM, Lubbers EJ, Kuijpers JH. Postoperative and long-term results of ileal pouch-anal anastomosis for ulcerative colitis and familial polyposis coli. Dig Dis Sci. 1992;37:1882–9.
79. Shepherd NA, Healey CD, Warren BE, et al. Distribution of mucosal pathology and an assessment of colonic phenotypic change in the pelvic ileal reservoir. Gut. 1993;34:101–5.
80. Kmiot WA, Youngs D, Tudor R, et al. Mucosal morphology, cell proliferation and faecal bacteriology in acute pouchitis. Br J Surg. 1993;80:1445–9.
81. Duffy M, O'Mahony L, Coffey JC, et al. Sulfate-reducing bacteria colonize pouches formed for ulcerative colitis but not for familial adenomatous polyposis. Dis Colon Rectum. 2002;45:384–8.
82. Bath S, Selinger CP, Leong RWL. The pathogenesis of primary pouchitis following ileal pouch-anal anastomosis: a review of current hypotheses. J Gastroenterol. 2011;1:7–12.
83. Ruseler-Van Embden JG, Schouten WR, van Lieshout LM. Pouchitis: result of microbial imbalance? Gut. 1994;35:658–64.
84. Tannock GW, Lawley B, Munro K, et al. Comprehensive analysis of the bacterial content of stool from patients with chronic pouchitis, normal pouches, or familial adenomatous polyposis pouches. Inflamm Bowel Dis. 2012;18:925–34.
85. Bambury N, Coffey JC, Burke J, et al. Sulphomucin expression in ileal pouches: emerging differences between ulcerative colitis and familial adenomatous polyposis pouches. Dis Colon Rectum. 2008;51:561–7.
86. Fumery M, Dulai PS, Meirick P, et al. Systematic review with meta-analysis: recurrence of Crohn's disease after total colectomy with permanent ileostomy. Aliment Pharmacol Ther. 2017;45:381–90.
87. Rutgeerts P, Goboes K, Peeters M, et al. Effect of faecal stream diversion on recurrence of Crohn's disease in the neoterminal ileum. Lancet. 1991;338:771–4.
88. D'Haens GR, Geboes K, Peeters M, et al. Early lesions of recurrent Crohn's disease caused by infusion of intestinal contents in excluded ileum. Gastroenterology. 1998;114:262–7.
89. Buisson A, Chevaux JB, Allen PB, et al. Review article: the natural history of postoperative Crohn's disease recurrence. Aliment Pharmacol Ther. 2012;35:625–33.
90. Shamah S, Schneider J, Korelitz BI. High incidence of recurrent Crohn's disease following colectomy for ulcerative colitis revealed with long follow-up. Dig Dis Sci. 2018;63:446–51.
91. Du P, Sun C, Ashburn J, et al. Risk factors for Crohn's disease of the neo-small intestine in ulcerative colitis patients with total proctocolectomy and primary or secondary ileostomies. J Crohns Colitis. 2015;9:170–6.
92. Koriche D, Gower-Rousseau C, Chater C, et al. Post-operative recurrence of Crohn's disease after definitive stoma: an underestimated risk. Int J Color Dis. 2017;32:453–8.
93. Nessar G, Fazio VW, Tekkis P, et al. Long-term outcome and quality of life after continent ileostomy. Dis Colon Rectum. 2006;49:336–44.
94. Handelsman JC, Gottlieb LM, Hamilton SR. Crohn's disease as a contraindication to Kock pouch (continent ileostomy). Dis Colon Rectum. 1993;36:840–3.
95. Brown CJ, Maclean AR, Cohen Z, et al. Crohn's disease and indeterminate colitis and the ileal pouch-anal anastomosis: outcomes and patterns of failure. Dis Colon Rectum. 2005;48:1542–9.
96. Gemlo BT, Wong WD, Rothenberger DA, Goldberg SM. Ileal pouch-anal anastomosis. Patterns of failure. Arch Surg. 1992;127:784–7.
97. Fazio VW, Ziv Y, Church JM, et al. Ileal pouch-anal anastomosis: complications and function in 1005 patients. Ann Surg. 1995;222:120–7.
98. Neilly P, Neill ME, Hill GL. Restorative proctocolectomy with ileal pouch-anal anastomosis in 203 patients: the Auckland experience. Aust NZ J Surg. 1999;69:22–7.
99. Keighley MRB. The final diagnosis in pouch patients for presumed ulcerative colitis may change to Crohn's disease: patients should be warned of the consequences. Acta Chir Ingoslav. 2000;47(suppl 4):27–31.
100. Yu CS, Pemberton JH, Larson D. Ileal pouch-anal anastomosis in patients with indeterminate colitis: long-term results. Dis Colon Rectum. 2000;43:1487–96.

101. Peyrègne V, Francois Y, Gilly FN, Descos JL, Flourie B, Vignal J. Outcome of ileal pouch after secondary diagnosis of Crohn's disease. Int J Color Dis. 2000;15:49–53.
102. Tulchinsky H, Hawley PR, Nicholls J. Long-term failure after restorative proctocolectomy for ulcerative colitis. Ann Surg. 2003;238:229–34.
103. Hartley JE, Fazio VW, Remzi FH, et al. Analysis of the outcome of ileal pouch-anal anastomosis in patients with Crohn's disease. Dis Colon Rectum. 2004;47:1808–15.
104. Murrell ZA, Melmed GY, Ippoliti A, et al. A prospective evaluation of the long-term outcome of ileal pouch-anal anastomosis in patients with inflammatory bowel disease-unclassified and indeterminate colitis. Dis Colon Rectum. 2009;52:872–8.
105. Delaney CP, Remzi FH, Gramlich T, et al. Equivalent function, quality of life and pouch survival rates after ileal pouch-anal anastomosis for indeterminate and ulcerative colitis. Ann Surg. 2002;236:43–8.
106. Melmed GY, Fleshner PR, Bardakcioglu O, et al. Family history and serology predict Crohn's disease after ileal pouch-anal anastomosis for ulcerative colitis. Dis Colon Rectum. 2008;51:100–8.
107. Shen B, Remzi FH, Hammel JP, et al. Family history of Crohn's disease increases the risk for Crohn's disease of ileal pouch-anal anastomosis. Inflamm Bowel Dis. 2009;15:163–70.
108. Stahlberg D, Gullberg K, Liljeqvist L, et al. Pouchitis following pelvic pouch operation for ulcerative colitis. Incidence, cumulative risk, and risk factors. Dis Colon Rectum. 1996;39:1012–8.
109. Hata K, Watanabe T, Shinozaki M, Nagawa H. Patients with extraintestinal manifestations have a higher risk of developing pouchitis in ulcerative colitis: multivariate analysis. Scand J Gastroenterol. 2003;38:1055–8.
110. Wasmuth HH, Svinsås M, Tranø G, et al. Surgical load and long-term outcome for patients with Kock continent ileostomy. Color Dis. 2007;9:713–7.
111. Köhler LW, Pemberton JH, Zinsmeister AR, Kelly KA. Quality of life after proctocolectomy. A comparison of Brooke ileostomy, Kock pouch, and ileal pouch-anal anastomosis. Gastroenterology. 1991;101:679–84.
112. Crawshaw A, Williams J, Woodhouse F. The Kock pouch reconsidered: an alternative surgical technique. Br J Nurs. 2014;23:S26–9.
113. Taleban S, Van Oijen MG, Vasiliauskas EA, et al. Colectomy with permanent end ileostomy is more cost-effective than ileal pouch-anal anastomosis for Crohn's colitis. Dig Dis Sci. 2016;61:550–9.
114. Dehni N, Remacle G, Dozois RR, et al. Salvage reoperation for complications after ileal pouch-anal anastomosis. Br J Surg. 2005;92:748–53.
115. Baixauli J, Delaney CP, Wu JS, et al. Functional outcome and quality of life after repeat ileal pouchanal anastomosis for complications of ileoanal surgery. Dis Colon Rectum. 2004;47:2–11.
116. Baert F, Moortgat L, Van Assche G, et al. Mucosal healing predicts sustained clinical remission in patients with early-stage Crohn's disease. Gastroenterology. 2010;138:463–8.
117. Colombel JF, Narula N, Peyrin-Biroulet L. Management strategies to improve outcomes of patients with inflammatory bowel diseases. Gastroenterology. 2017;152:351–61.
118. Colombel JF, Sandborn WJ, Reinisch W, et al. Infliximab, azathioprine, or combination therapy for Crohn's disease. N Engl J Med. 2010;362:1383–95.
119. D'Haens G, Baert F, van Assche G, et al. Early combined immunosuppression or conventional management in patients with newly diagnosed Crohn's disease: an open randomised trial. Lancet. 2008;371:660–7.
120. Colombel JF, Reinisch W, Mantzaris GJ, et al. Randomised clinical trial: deep remission in biologic and immunomodulator naive patients with Crohn's disease - a SONIC post hoc analysis. Aliment Pharmacol Ther. 2015;41:734–46.
121. Colombel JF, Sandborn WJ, Rutgeerts P, et al. Adalimumab for maintenance of clinical response and remission in patients with Crohn's disease: the CHARM trial. Gastroenterology. 2007;132:52–65.

122. Silverberg MS, Satsangi J, Ahmad T, et al. Toward an integrated clinical, molecular and sero-logical classification of inflammatory bowel disease: report of a working party of the 2005 Montreal world congress of gastroenterology. Can J Gastroenterol. 2005;19(Suppl A):5–36.
123. Satsangi J, Silverberg MS, Vermeire S, et al. The Montreal classification of inflammatory bowel disease: controversies, consensus, and implications. Gut. 2006;55:749–53.
124. Shen B, Remzi FH, Lavery IC, et al. A proposed classification of ileal pouch disorders and associated complications after restorative proctocolectomy for ulcerative colitis. Clin Gastroenterol Hepatol. 2008;6:145–58.
125. Orscheln ES, Dillman JR, Towbin AJ, et al. Penetrating Crohn disease: does it occur in the absence of stricturing disease? Abdom Radiol (NY). 2017.; [Epub ahead of print]
126. Abdelrazeq AS, Kelly SM, Lund JN, Leveson SH. Rifaximin-ciprofloxacin combination therapy is effective in chronic active refractory pouchitis. Color Dis. 2005;7:182.
127. Shen B, Remzi FH, Lopez AR, Queener E. Rifaximin for maintenance therapy in antibiotic-dependent pouchitis. BMC Gastroenterol. 2008;8:26.
128. Kelly OB, Rosenberg M, Tyler AD, et al. Infliximab to treat refractory inflammation after pelvic pouch surgery for ulcerative colitis. J Crohns Colitis. 2016;10:410–7.
129. Huguet M, Pereira B, Goutte M, et al. Systematic review with meta-analysis: anti-TNF therapy in refractory pouchitis and Crohn's disease-like complications of the pouch ffter ileal pouch-anal anastomosis following colectomy for ulcerative colitis. Inflamm Bowel Dis. 2018;24:261–8.
130. Bär F, Kühbacher T, Dietrich NA, et al. German IBD study group. Vedolizumab in the treat-ment of chronic, antibiotic-dependent or refractory pouchitis. Aliment Pharmacol Ther. 2018;47:581–7.
131. Verstockt B, Claeys C, Van Assche G, et al. Vedolizumab can induce clinical remission in patients with chronic antibiotic-refractory pouchitis: A retrospective single-centre experi-ence. The ECCO congress, Vienna 2018, abstract P624.
132. Rezaie A, Kuenzig ME, Benchimol EI, et al. Budesonide for induction of remission in Crohn's disease. Cochrane Database Syst Rev. 2015;6:CD000296.
133. Greenberg GR, Feagan BG, Martin F, et al. Oral budesonide for active Crohn's disease. Canadian inflammatory bowel disease study group. N Engl J Med. 1994;331:836–41.
134. Rutgeerts P, Lofberg R, Malchow H, et al. A comparison of budesonide with prednisolone for active Crohn's disease. N Engl J Med. 1994;331:842–5.
135. Campieri M, Ferguson A, Doe W, et al. Oral budesonide is as effective as oral prednisolone in active Crohn's disease. The global budesonide study group. Gut. 1997;41:209–14.
136. Bar-Meir S, Chowers Y, Lavy A, et al. Budesonide versus prednisone in the treatment of active Crohn's disease. The Israeli budesonide study group. Gastroenterology. 1998;115:835–40.
137. Benchimol EI, Seow CH, Steinhart AH, et al. Traditional corticosteroids for induction of remission in Crohn's disease. Cochrane Database Syst Rev. 2008:CD006792.
138. Schoon EJ, Bollani S, Mills PR, et al. Bone mineral density in relation to efficacy and side effects of budesonide and prednisolone in Crohn's disease. Clin Gastroenterol Hepatol. 2005;3:113–21.
139. Lichtenstein GR, Feagan BG, Cohen RD, et al. Serious infection and mortality in patients with Crohn's disease: more than 5 years of follow-up in the TREAT registry. Am J Gastroenterol. 2012;107:1409–22.
140. Toruner M, Loftus EV Jr, Harmsen WS, et al. Risk factors for opportunistic infections in patients with inflammatory bowel disease. Gastroenterology. 2008;134:929–36.
141. Kuenzig ME, Rezaie A, Seow CH, et al. Budesonide for maintenance of remission in Crohn's disease. Cochrane Database Syst Rev. 2014;8:CD002913.298.
142. Steinhart AH, Ewe K, Griffiths AM, et al. Corticosteroids for maintenance of remission in Crohn's disease. Cochrane Database Syst Rev. 2003:CD000301.
143. Summers RW, Switz DM, Sessions JT, et al. National cooperative Crohn's disease study: results of drug treatment. Gastroenterology. 1979;77:847–69.
144. Malchow H, Ewe K, Brandes JW, et al. European cooperative Crohn's disease study (ECCDS): results of drug treatment. Gastroenterology. 1984;86:249–66.

145. Munkholm P, Langholz E, Davidsen M, Binder V. Frequency of glucocorticoid resistance and dependency in Crohn's disease. Gut. 1994;35:360–2.
146. Faubion WA Jr, Loftus EV Jr, Harmsen WS, et al. The natural history of corticosteroid therapy for inflammatory bowel disease: a population-based study. Gastroenterology. 2001;121:255–60.
147. Ho GT, Chiam P, Drummond H, et al. The efficacy of corticosteroid therapy in inflammatory bowel disease: analysis of a 5-year UK inception cohort. Aliment Pharmacol Ther. 2006;24:319–30.
148. Colombel JF, Panaccione R, Bossuyt P, et al. Effect of tight control management on Crohn's disease (CALM): a multicentre, randomised, controlled phase 3 trial. Lancet. 2018;390:2779–89.
149. Colombel JF, Reinisch W, Mantzaris GJ, et al. Randomised clinical trial: deep remission in biologic and immunomodulator naïve patients with Crohn's disease - a SONIC post hoc analysis. Aliment Pharmacol Ther. 2015;41:734–46.
150. Present DH, Korelitz BI, Wisch N, et al. Treatment of Crohn's disease with 6-mercaptopurine. A long-term, randomized, double-blind study. N Engl J Med. 1980;302:981–7.
151. Prefontaine E, Macdonald JK, Sutherland LR. Azathioprine or 6-mercaptopurine for induction of remission in Crohn's disease. Cochrane Database Syst Rev. 2010;6:CD000545.
152. Chande N, Townsend CM, Parker CE, MacDonald JK. Azathioprine or 6-mercaptopurine for induction of remission in Crohn's disease. Cochrane Database Syst Rev. 2016;10:CD000545.
153. Chande N, Patton PH, Tsoulis DJ, et al. Azathioprine or 6-mercaptopurine for maintenance of remission in Crohn's disease. Cochrane Database Syst Rev. 2015;10:CD000067.
154. de Boer NKH, Peyrin-Biroulet L, Jharap B, et al. Thiopurines in inflammatory bowel disease: new findings and perspectives. J Crohns Colitis. 2017. [Epub ahead of print].
155. Louis E, Mary JY, Vernier-Massouille G, et al. Maintenance of remission among patients with Crohn's disease on antimetabolite therapy after infliximab therapy is stopped. Gastroenterology. 2012;142:63–70.
156. Van Asseldonk DP, de Boer NK, Peters GJ, et al. On therapeutic drug monitoring of thiopurines in inflammatory bowel disease; pharmacology, pharmacogenomics, drug intolerance and clinical relevance. Curr Drug Metab. 2009;10:981–97.
157. Jharap B, Seinen ML, de Boer NK, et al. Thiopurine therapy in inflammatory bowel disease patients: analyses of two 8-year intercept cohorts. Inflamm Bowel Dis. 2010;16:1541–9.
158. Coenen MJ, de Jong DJ, van Marrewijk CJ, et al. Identification of patients with variants in TPMT and dose reduction reduces hematologic events during thiopurine treatment of inflammatory bowel disease. Gastroenterology. 2015;149:907–17.
159. Dubinsky MC, Lamothe S, Yang HY, et al. Pharmacogenomics and metabolite measurement for 6-mercaptopurine therapy in inflammatory bowel disease. Gastroenterology. 2000;118:705–13.
160. Yarur AJ, Gondal B, Hirsch A, et al. Higher thioguanine nucleotide metabolite levels are associated with better long-term outcomes in patients with inflammatory bowel diseases. J Clin Gastroenterol. 2017. [Epub ahead of print].
161. Dubinsky MC, Yang H, Hassard PV, et al. 6-MP metabolite profiles provide a biochemical explanation for 6-MP resistance in patients with inflammatory bowel disease. Gastroenterology. 2002;122:904–15.
162. Ansari A, Patel N, Sanderson J, et al. Low-dose azathioprine or mercaptopurine in combination with allopurinol can bypass many adverse drug reactions in patients with inflammatory bowel disease. Aliment Pharmacol Ther. 2010;31:640–7.
163. Sparrow MP. Use of allopurinol to optimize thiopurine immunomodulator efficacy in inflammatory bowel disease. Gastroenterol Hepatol (N Y). 2008;4:505–11.
164. Nagy F, Molnar T, Szepes Z, et al. Efficacy of 6-mercaptopurine treatment after azathioprine hypersensitivity in inflammatory bowel disease. World J Gastroenterol. 2008;14:4342–6.
165. Bermejo F, Lopez-Sanroman A, Algaba A, et al. Mercaptopurine rescue after azathioprine-induced liver injury in inflammatory bowel disease. Aliment Pharmacol Ther. 2010;31:120–4.

166. Herfarth HH, Kappelman MD, Long MD, et al. Use of methotrexate in the treatment of inflammatory bowel diseases. Inflamm Bowel Dis. 2016;22:224–33.
167. Feagan BG, Rochon J, Fedorak RN, et al. Methotrexate for the treatment of Crohn's disease. The north American Crohn's study group investigators. N Engl J Med. 1995;332:292–7.
168. McDonald JW, Wang Y, Tsoulis DJ, et al. Methotrexate for induction of remission in refractory Crohn's disease. Cochrane Database Syst Rev. 2014;8:CD003459.
169. Feagan BG, Fedorak RN, Irvine EJ, et al. A comparison of methotrexate with placebo for the maintenance of remission in Crohn's disease. North American Crohn's study group investigators. N Engl J Med. 2000;342:1627–32.
170. Patel V, Wang Y, MacDonald JK, et al. Methotrexate for maintenance of remission in Crohn's disease. Cochrane Database Syst Rev. 2014;8:CD006884.
171. Kurnik D, Loebstein R, Fishbein E, et al. Bioavailability of oral vs. subcutaneous low-dose methotrexate in patients with Crohn's disease. Aliment Pharmacol Ther. 2003;18:57–63.
172. Sokol H, Seksik P, Carrat F, et al. Usefulness of co-treatment with immunomodulators in patients with inflammatory bowel disease treated with scheduled infliximab maintenance therapy. Gut. 2010;59:1363–8.
173. Yarur AJ, Kubiliun MJ, Czul F, et al. Concentrations of 6-thioguanine nucleotide correlate with trough levels of infliximab in patients with inflammatory bowel disease on combination therapy. Clin Gastroenterol Hepatol. 2015;13:1118–24.
174. Roblin X, Boschetti G, Williet N, et al. Azathioprine dose reduction in inflammatory bowel disease patients on combination therapy: an open-label, prospective and randomised clinical trial. Aliment Pharmacol Ther. 2017;46:142–9.
175. Ungar B, Kopylov U, Engel T, et al. Addition of an immunomodulator can reverse antibody formation and loss of response in patients treated with adalimumab. Aliment Pharmacol Ther. 2017;45:276–82.
176. Ben-Horin S, Waterman M, Kopylov U, et al. Addition of an immunomodulator to infliximab therapy eliminates antidrug antibodies in serum and restores clinical response of patients with inflammatory bowel disease. Clin Gastroenterol Hepatol. 2013;11:444–7.
177. Bots S, Gecse K, Barclay M, D'Haens G. Combination Immunosuppression in IBD. Inflamm Bowel Dis. 2018;24:539–45.
178. Lemaitre M, Kirchgesner J, Rudnichi A, et al. Association between use of thiopurines or tumor necrosis factor antagonists alone or in combination and risk of lymphoma in patients with inflammatory bowel disease. JAMA. 2017;318:1679–86.
179. Osterman MT, Haynes K, Delzell E, et al. Effectiveness and safety of immunomodulators with anti-tumor necrosis factor therapy in Crohn's disease. Clin Gastroenterol Hepatol. 2015;13:1293–301.
180. Sandborn WJ, Feagan BG, Rutgeerts P, et al. Vedolizumab as induction and maintenance therapy for Crohn's disease. N Engl J Med. 2013;369:711–21.
181. Sands BE, Feagan BG, Rutgeerts P, et al. Effects of vedolizumab induction therapy for patients with Crohn's disease in whom tumor necrosis factor antagonist treatment failed. Gastroenterology. 2014;147:618–27.
182. Sandborn WJ, Feagan BG, Fedorak RN, et al. A randomized trial of Ustekinumab, a human interleukin-12/23 monoclonal antibody, in patients with moderate-to-severe Crohn's disease. Gastroenterology. 2008;135:1130–41.
183. Yarur AJ, Rubin DT. Therapeutic drug monitoring of anti-tumor necrosis factor agents in patients with inflammatory bowel diseases. Inflamm Bowel Dis. 2015;21:1709–18.
184. Ben-Horin S. Drug level-based anti-tumor necrosis factor therapy: ready for prime time? Gastroenterology. 2015;148:1268–71.
185. Mitrev N, Leong RW. Therapeutic drug monitoring of anti-tumour necrosis factor-α agents in inflammatory bowel disease. Expert Opin Drug Saf. 2017;16:303–17.
186. Hassan C, Zullo A, De Francesco V, et al. Systematic review: endoscopic dilatation in Crohn's disease. Aliment Pharmacol Ther. 2007;26:1457–64.

187. Shen B, Fazio VW, Remzi FH, et al. Endoscopic balloon dilation of ileal pouch strictures. Am J Gastroenterol. 2004;99:2340–7.
188. Reese GE, Purkayastha S, Tilney HS, et al. Strictureplasty vs resection in small bowel Crohn's disease: an evaluation of short-term outcomes and recurrence. Color Dis. 2007;9:686–94.
189. Yamamoto T, Fazio VW, Tekkis PP. Safety and efficacy of strictureplasty for crohn's disease: a systematic review and meta-analysis. Dis Colon Rectum. 2007;50:1968–86.
190. Fearnhead NS, Chowdhury R, Box B, et al. Long-term follow-up of strictureplasty for Crohn's disease. Br J Surg. 2006;93:475–82.
191. Matzke GM, Kang AS, Dozois EJ, et al. Mid pouch stricturoplasty for Crohn's disease after ileal pouch-anal anastomosis: an alternative to pouch excision. Dis Colon Rectum. 2004;47:782–6.
192. Wu XR, Mukewar S, Kiran RP, et al. Surgical stricturoplasty in the treatment of ileal pouch strictures. J Gastrointest Surg. 2013;17:1452–61.
193. Sagar PM, Dozois RR, Wolff BG. Long-term results of ileal pouch-anal anastomosis in patients with Crohn's disease. Dis Colon Rectum. 1996;39:893–8.
194. Present DH, Rutgeerts P, Targan S, et al. Infliximab for the treatment of fistulas in patients with Crohn's disease. N Engl J Med. 1999;340:1398–405.
195. Sands BE, Anderson FH, Bernstein CN, Chey WY, Feagan BG, Fedorak RN, et al. Infliximab maintenance therapy for fistulizing Crohn's disease. N Engl J Med. 2004;350(9):876–85.
196. Sands BE, Blank MA, Patel K, et al. Long-term treatment of rectovaginal fistulas in Crohn's disease: response to infliximab in the ACCENT II study. Clin Gastroenterol Hepatol. 2004;2:912–20.
197. Colombel JF, Schwartz DA, Sandborn WJ, et al. Adalimumab for the treatment of fistulas in patients with Crohn's disease. Gut. 2009;58:940–8.
198. Gecse KB, Bemelman W, Kamm MA, et al. A global consensus on the classification, diagnosis and multidisciplinary treatment of perianal fistulising Crohn's disease. Gut. 2014;63:1381–92.
199. Molendijk I, Peeters KC, Baeten CI, et al. Improving the outcome of fistulising Crohn's disease. Best Pract Res Clin Gastroenterol. 2014;28:505–18.
200. Pearson DC, May GR, Fick GH, Sutherland LR. Azathioprine and 6-mercaptopurine in Crohn disease. A meta-analysis. Ann Intern Med. 1995;123:132–42.
201. Gionchetti P, Dignass A, Danese S, et al. 3rd European evidence-based consensus on the diagnosis and Management of Crohn's disease 2016: part 2: surgical management and special situations. J Crohns Colitis. 2017;11:135–49.
202. West RL, van der Woude CJ, Hansen BE, et al. Clinical and endosonographic effect of ciprofloxacin on the treatment of perianal fistulae in Crohn's disease with infliximab: a double-blind placebo-controlled study. Aliment Pharmacol Ther. 2004;20:1329–36.
203. Dewint P, Hansen BE, Verhey E, et al. Adalimumab combined with ciprofloxacin is superior to adalimumab monotherapy in perianal fistula closure in Crohn's disease: a randomised, double-blind, placebo controlled trial (ADAFI). Gut. 2014;63:292–9.

Chapter 16
Quality of Life and the Continent Ileostomy

Tom Øresland

16.1 Introduction

During the 1950s and 60s the golden standard treatment for patients with Ulcerative Colitis was a proctocolectomy with an end-ileostomy. After it had been clearly demonstrated by Truelove and Witts in the mid-1950s that early surgery in severe colitis not responding to steroids was a life-saving procedure, acute fulminant or severe colitis was no longer associated with death rates in the range of 20–40%. Thus more patients survived and with the increase in incidence rates more people were left with an end-ileostomy. It was about this time that Brian Brooke demonstrated that eversion of the protruding stoma with a mucocutaneous suturing of the bowel to the skin made life with a stoma becoming almost bearable for a majority of patients. Still, life with an end-ileostomy was mostly a sentence to life in isolation with very few social contacts and severe practical problems with stoma dressing, skin erosion, leakage of bowel content and foul smell. Bear in mind that the people affected was mostly young not having found a partner. Modern stoma appliances as we know them today were first introduced in a large scale in the early 1970ties.

It was in this setting that Nils G. Kock was working and he was very much aware of these problems. The development of the continent ileostomy was driven purely for the purpose of providing patients a better quality of life. Kock was a surgeon devoted to the quality of life of his patients and this drove him through the many steps of developing the continent ileostomy as we know it today. One of his first patients was a nurse and she was trained at the Cleveland Clinic to become the first Scandinavian enterostoma therapist. Having a solid backup in terms of

T. Øresland (✉)
Institute of Clinical Medicine, University of Oslo and Department of GI surgery, Akershus University Hospital, Lørenskog, Norway
e-mail: tom.oresland@medisin.uio.no

© Springer Nature Switzerland AG 2019
P. Myrelid, M. Block (eds.), *The Kock Pouch*,
https://doi.org/10.1007/978-3-319-95591-9_16

enterostoma therapists and a qualified team around the patient is crucial for success and a good quality of life. As is also pointed out in other chapters of this book, selecting and informing patients before surgery is mandatory and a prerequisite for a good outcome.

16.2   Functional Aspects

When functioning as intended the continent ileostomy gives in comparison to the end-ileostomy an excellent quality of life. The stoma is placed below the belt line and when deciding the stoma site one does not have to take into consideration the quality of the surrounding skin with respect to the fitting of a stoma appliance. The only requisite is that it should be possible to apply a gauze pad. Thus it is easier to hide the continent stoma with minimal clothing and the other advantage with respect to quality of life is that it does not protrude above the skin level. For patients with an established continent ileostomy it is recommended that the pouch is intubated three to five times daily although there are those who will empty both more and less frequent. One should be aware that the semi-fluid bowel content is only a part of what's harbored within the pouch for some patients as the amount of gas is equal to or even higher than the fluid. On average the fecal content is about 700 ml whereas the gas constitutes up to 1500 ml. Thus the reason for this recommendation to empty four times daily is the belief that an overfilled pouch will put strain on the attachment to the anterior abdominal wall and thus it might be a first step in nipple valve slippage.

As the continent ileostomy is not leaking any gases it does not give any foul smell. The amount of gas is most probably dependent not only on the diet but also on how much air that is swallowed and the variability is great. When gas is a problem patients should have this information. Also some people have a rather solid content in the pouch besides the gas and they need to flush the pouch with tap water before emptying. Another functional aspect which to some extent is not so prominent in the pelvic pouch situation is the fact that the continent ileostomy patients usually have their rectums excised. In females this will alter the gross anatomy in the pelvis in that the vagina will fall back get angulated and maybe there will be dense adhesions formed against the pelvis. This impairs the natural drainage of the vagina and can give rise to excess vaginal discharge. The angulation and adhesions might also give sexual dysfunction with dyspareunia. Furthermore, adhesions in the pelvis affecting the fallopian tubes will negatively influence fecundity, i.e. the ability to be pregnant through intercourse. Occluded fallopian tubes can be seen in 50% of women who have had their rectum excised. However, this and the possible nerve damage inflicted during the pelvic dissection is also a problem when replacing the rectum with an ileal pouch-anal anastomosis.

16.3 Quality of Life

There are several testimonies to the improved quality of life with a continent ileostomy. The best proof is by the patients themselves. Once having experienced a well-functioning Kock pouch they are very reluctant to give it up when there are problems with the Kock pouch. Most patients will gladly submit to numerous re-operations with revisions of the pouch. Sometimes not to say rather frequently it is the surgeon who has to say no and stop further revision attempts. Some patients do not form adhesions and those are probably most at risk for multiple revisions.

However, when the nipple valve is not working as intended the patients will have leakage which is particularly distressing since the stoma is flush with the skin and situated where conventional appliances might not perform very well. Furthermore valve slippage is distressing in that it might incur that intubation of the pouch becomes increasingly difficult. Since many patients will experience this it must be included in the total lifelong quality of life equation.

The individual's perception of quality of life is dependent on their life situation at large, social interactions, self-esteem, and life conditions in general. However, when assessing quality of life after surgery the pre-operative status is also of concern. Those having suffered heavily over time with a considerable symptom burden tend to appreciate the results of surgery more than those where the operation was mandated by risk of developing a cancer. Despite equal post-operative functioning the former group tends to perceive their quality of life as better.

The early reports on the continent ileostomy and quality of life highlighted the absence of skin problems and odor. Less time spent with stoma care, clothing worn more comfortably increasing confidence during sports, on social occasions and in sexual relations. From countries where the patients have to pay for stoma care themselves it was also pointed out that the continent ileostomy reduces costs dramatically. A later study on patients with long term follow-up of median 30 years reported that patients evacuate a median of four times a day. Some 18% experienced leakage and a 10% had skin problems. Seventy eight percent rated their health as good to excellent and as in most studies the Short Form 36 health surveys was comparable to reference values. It should be noted that these patients were operated during the time period when the technique was still under development, thus they may not compare to patients operated in more recent years. A further study on how these patients adjusted to daily life revealed that the quality and availability of public restrooms posed a problem. Having to remove the continent ileostomy and revert to an end-ileostomy is shown to diminish quality of life in a wide range of aspects.

Comparisons between an end-ileostomy, a continent ileostomy and a pelvic pouch were first made by Köhler et al. It was shown that the patients with pelvic pouch had fewer restrictions in sports and sexual activities than those with a continent ileostomy. Patients with a continent ileostomy had in turn fewer restrictions in these activities, but more restrictions in travelling, than patients with an end-ileostomy.

Patients who have had their pelvic pouch converted to a continent ileostomy can also expect to have the same quality of life advantages as those who have had a primary Kock pouch. The results in a pediatric population seem no different but it is advised a rigid selection and that no patients younger than teenage should receive this pouch.

16.4 Sexual Function

A survey in the early 1980s of sexual adjustment in end-ileostomy patients before and after conversion to a continent ileostomy revealed that most patients had felt embarrassed with their conventional stoma whereas only 24% had these reactions after conversion to a Kock pouch. Also their partners reported that they in contrary to the conventional stoma had no negative reactions towards the continent ileostomy. Conversion to a continent ileostomy improved the quality of sexual life in about 85% of both women and men. It is also to expect normal pregnancies and deliveries in patients with a continent ileostomy. A cesarean is indicated only for obstetric or other reasons. In a few instances ileostomy function will be disturbed during the late phases of the pregnancy sometimes necessitating revision surgery.

Ostomy surgery influences multiple aspects of the Islamic religious practice. Perception of cleanliness is central to some of these activities. One might speculate that a continent ileostomy perhaps would be a better alternative for religious Muslims with these aspects in mind.

16.5 General Aspects on Quality of Life

As relatively few continent ileostomies are constructed today, the population of people with continent ileostomies is getting older. Some will have dementia and will not be able to care for themselves. Thus it is important that knowledge about the continent ileostomy is maintained in the medical society. This is not an easy task and it has happened more than once that an elderly patient has been admitted to hospital for whatever reason and the young doctor has noted a stoma but without the appliance. A stoma bag has been ordered and some hours or even days later it is noted that nothing is produced and the abdomen seems a bit distended. The radical solution that might perhaps be the only secure solution is to have a tattoo above the stoma informing that it is continent and has to be intubated.

The now emerging referral clinics in the area of inflammatory bowel disease with multidisciplinary teams should provide a safe haven for the small group of patients with a continent ileostomy. Quality of life is much dependent on feeling secure knowing that there is expertise around you. The provision of good quality of care in chronic diseases requires an approach with greater access to information for patients, education and empowerment. In this process, a key role for enterostoma therapists and inflammatory bowel disease specialty nurses is increasingly recognized.

16.6   Specific Problems Affecting Quality of Life

Pouchitis is a well-known problem affecting the pelvic pouch, actually first described in continent ileostomies by Nils G. Kock himself. The incidence is seemingly a bit lower than in the pelvic pouch. It might be that the nipple valve protects against modest symptoms of pouchitis in a way that is not possible in the pelvic pouch, where continence is more relative and dependent on the status of the anal canal and the anal sphincter. Local treatment of inflammation of the continent ileostomy can easily be achieved by introducing a suppository e.g. metronidazole into the pouch after emptying. Still having an increased output perhaps with some blood and in the worst of cases with abdominal pain will negatively affect quality of life in patients with a continent ileostomy.

Mucous secretion from the nipple valve and outlet bowel poses a problem in some patients mostly it is well contained in the dressing and of no big consequence. Some patients do have more problems and have to change the stoma gauze more often than emptying frequency indicates. Local anesthetics like lidocaine gel introduced into the valve have been used to alleviate this but there is no good documentation on the efficacy.

Bibliography

1. Truelove SC, Witts LJ. Cortisone in ulcerative colitis; final report on a therapeutic trial. Br Med J. 1955;2(4947):1041–8.
2. Brooke BN. The management of an ileostomy, including its complications. Lancet. 1952;2(6725):102–4.
3. Brevinge H, Berglund B, Kock NG. Ileostomy output of gas and feces before and after conversion from conventional to reservoir ileostomy. Dis Colon Rectum. 1992;35(7):662–9.
4. Oresland T, Palmblad S, Ellstrom M, Berndtsson I, Crona N, Hulten L. Gynaecological and sexual function related to anatomical changes in the female pelvis after restorative proctocolectomy. Int J Color Dis. 1994;9(2):77–81.
5. Gerber A, Apt MK, Craig PH. The improved quality of life with the Kock continent ileostomy. J Clin Gastroenterol. 1984;6(6):513–7.
6. Berndtsson IE, Lindholm E, Oresland T, Hulten L. Health-related quality of life and pouch function in continent ileostomy patients: a 30-year perspective. Dis Colon Rectum. 2004;47(12):2131–7.
7. Berndtsson I, Lindholm E, Ekman I. Thirty years of experience living with a continent ileostomy: bad restrooms--not my reservoir--decide my life. J Wound Ostomy Continence Nurs. 2005;32(5):321–6. quiz 327–328.
8. Nessar G, Fazio VW, Tekkis P, et al. Long-term outcome and quality of life after continent ileostomy. Dis Colon Rectum. 2006;49(3):336–44.
9. Kohler LW, Pemberton JH, Zinsmeister AR, Kelly KA. Quality of life after proctocolectomy. A comparison of Brooke ileostomy, Kock pouch, and ileal pouch-anal anastomosis. Gastroenterology. 1991;101(3):679–84.
10. Parc Y, Klouche M, Bennis M, Lefevre JH, Shields C, Tiret E. The continent ileostomy: an alternative to end ileostomy? Short and long-term results of a single institution series. Dig Liver Dis. 2011;43(10):779–83.

11. Lian L, Fazio VW, Remzi FH, Shen B, Dietz D, Kiran RP. Outcomes for patients undergoing continent ileostomy after a failed ileal pouch-anal anastomosis. Dis Colon Rectum. 2009;52(8):1409–14. discussion 4414-1406.
12. Ein SH. A ten-year experience with the pediatric Kock pouch. J Pediatr Surg. 1987;22(8):764–6.
13. Nilsson LO, Kock NG, Kylberg F, Myrvold HE, Palselius I. Sexual adjustment in ileostomy patients before and after conversion to continent ileostomy. Dis Colon Rectum. 1981;24(4):287–90.
14. Ojerskog B, Kock NG, Philipson BM, Philipson M. Pregnancy and delivery in patients with a continent ileostomy. Surg Gynecol Obstet. 1988;167(1):61–4.
15. Akgul B, Karadag A. The effect of colostomy and ileostomy on acts of worship in the Islamic faith. J Wound Ostomy Continence Nurs. 2016;43(4):392–7.
16. Svaninger G, Nordgren S, Oresland T, Hulten L. Incidence and characteristics of pouchitis in the Kock continent ileostomy and the pelvic pouch. Scand J Gastroenterol. 1993;28(8):695–700.

Chapter 17
Reoperations

Jonas Bengtson and Anna Solberg

17.1 Early Complications and Surgical Management

17.1.1 Ischemia

It is relatively common to see a certain degree of discolouring of the nipple mucosa after the stapling of the nipple. It may be caused by venous stasis leading to decreased arterial circulation as well and will most of the time solve itself. However, in the case of a more pronounced ischemia there is a risk of, if not a definite gangrene, for a later stricture of part or the whole nipple outlet.

If total ischemia is obvious during surgery the segment must be excised and a new nipple valve and outlet created, using the inlet or a more proximal segment of bowel above the inlet. These procedures are described in detail below.

In the case of a gangrene of the nipple valve in the early postoperative period, it is likewise necessary to make a resection of the segment, and if possible, save the remaining pouch for a later re-construction of the nipple valve and the outlet. This could be done by anchoring the pouch to the inside of the abdominal wall and to create a mucous fistula of the orifice of the excised nipple, and a defunctioning loop-ileostomy.

J. Bengtson (✉) · A. Solberg
Sahlgrenska University Hospital/Östra, Gothenburg, Sweden
e-mail: jonas.l.bengtsson@vgregion.se; anna.solberg@vgregion.se

© Springer Nature Switzerland AG 2019
P. Myrelid, M. Block (eds.), *The Kock Pouch*,
https://doi.org/10.1007/978-3-319-95591-9_17

17.2   Dehiscence of the Suture Lines or Catheter Associated Injury

Dehiscence of the suture lines (very uncommon) should be managed in the same way as for dehiscence in any anastomosis or suture lines. If it is possible to preserve the pouch it nearly always involves a proximal diversion. However, gangrene of the pouch prevent the possibility to pouch salvage. Leakage due to perforation of the catheter is equally rare and could be managed by proximal diversion.

17.3   Enterocutaneous Fistula

Early enterocutaneous fistula require drainage of the pouch as complete as possible including proximal diversion, with the hope of fistula healing and pouch preservation. An initial trial with nil by mouth and parenteral nutrition should be considered.

17.4   Revisional Surgery of the Kock Pouch

17.4.1   Optimizing the Patient

Optimal conditions for the patient includes the obvious; absence of sepsis, optimal nutritional status, long enough time since previous surgery, smoking cessation etc. For quite a few patients optimizing also means weight reduction as obesity is a risk factor per se and effectively could prevent optimal surgery, i.e. due to a fatty mesentery and/or a thick abdominal wall.

17.5   Nipple Valve Slippage

As has been shown in the previous chapters, the nipple valve is the Achilles heel of the construction and slipping of the nipple is also the most common indication for revisional surgery.

Slipping of the nipple is often, but not always, seen in combination with suboptimal anchoring of the pouch to the abdominal wall and/or widening of the opening through the abdominal wall, often obvious first at surgery.

Slipping of the nipple could be complete, but partial slipping to some degree, is probably more frequent. However, the mode of repair does not differ between a partial or complete des-invagination.

Consequently, after freeing the pouch, including the inlet, from adhesions the first step is to take down the pouch with the intact outlet from the abdominal wall. The pouch is then opened in a suture line to minimise the risk of creating areas with a sub optimal blood supply and a secondary ischemia. However, it is in some cases obvious from the beginning that the nipple valve could not be saved. Instead of opening the pouch with a separate incision, the defect after the excision of the nipple could be used for access to the pouch for further procedure.

It has been described to do a nipple repair without taking down the pouch from the abdominal wall. However, in our experience it is difficult to do as a complete repair as needed without a complete mobilisation of the pouch. There is a risk of missing, as previously mentioned, detachment of the pouch from the abdominal wall.

17.6   Re-Stapling

The first option to explore is the possibility of a re-stapling of the nipple. It is often feasible to remove the remaining staples to completely desuscept the nipple segment for the best opportunity to make a complete re-stapling, including a potential removal of excess fat from the mesentery.

It should also be considered to add stapling of the nipple to the pouch wall, either through the enterotomy or through a separate incision. Care should be taken to denude the mucosa from the nipple and the complementary area in the pouch (Figs. 17.1 and 17.2).

Fig. 17.1 Preparing the nipple valve for stapling to the pouch wall by denuding the mucosa

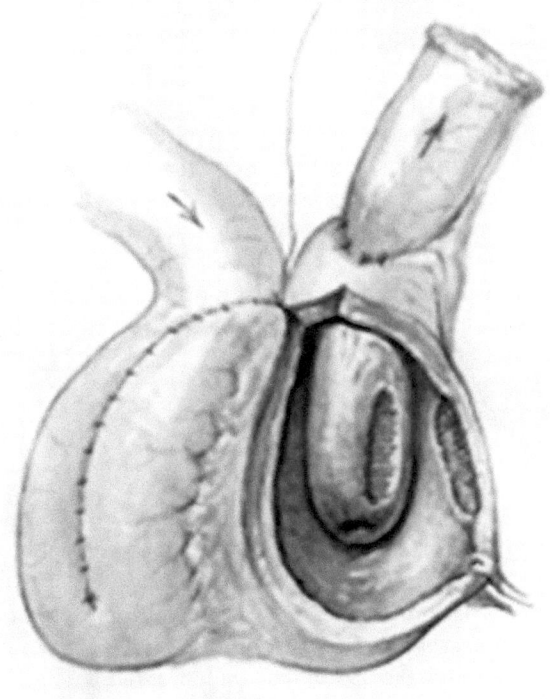

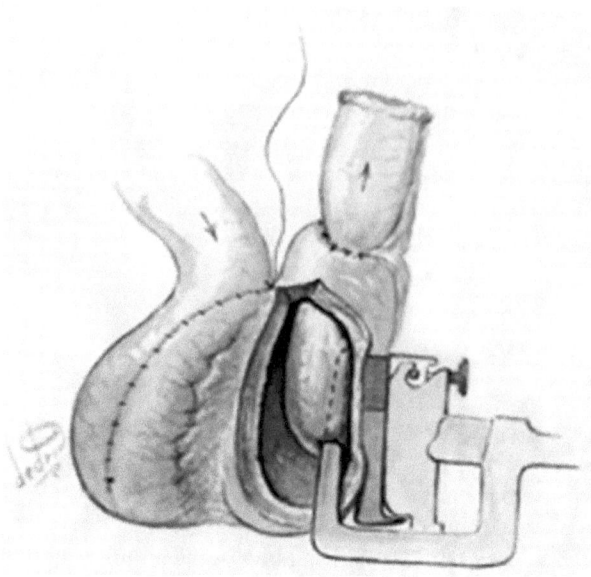

Fig. 17.2 Stapling the nipple valve to the pouch wall

17.7 Rotation of the Pouch

If the existing nipple can not be used for re-stapling due to impossibility to do the re-intussusception, damage to the nipple and/or blood supply during the dissection or a short outlet segment, the next option is to make an entirely new nipple of the pouch inlet. To make the opening after excision of the nipple and outlet as small as possible it could be of great help to reduce the invaginate to define the optimal resection line. The construction of the nipple valve is done in the same way as for a new constructed nipple. The proximal divided bowel is then anastomosed to the former outlet (Figs. 17.3, 17.4 and 17.5). Another option is of course to close the defect after the nipple excision and to anastomose the new inlet to a more suitable location if this facilitates the anchoring of the pouch to the abdominal wall.

17.8 Transposed Segment

There are also situations where the inlet could not be used, e.g. due to stricturing of the segment with or without dilatation of the proximal bowel. The option in that situation is to use a segment of bowel more proximal to the inlet. This segment should measure about 10 cm for the nipple and sufficient additional length for the outlet through the abdominal wall. The mesentery for the nipple is prepared in the same way as for a conventional or rotated nipple (Fig. 17.6). However, even more

Fig. 17.3 Outline of pouch rotation

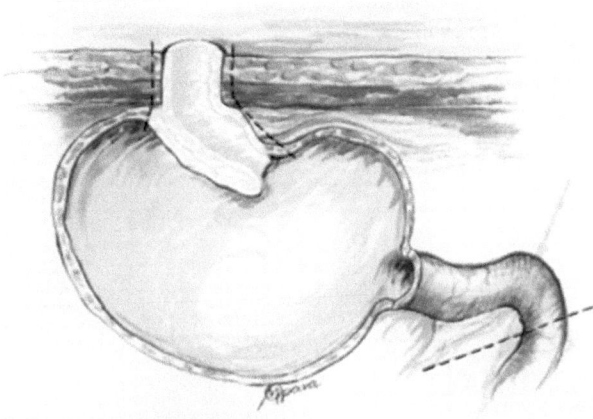

Fig. 17.4 The pouch inlet bowel used for the new nipple valve. Former nipple valve excised

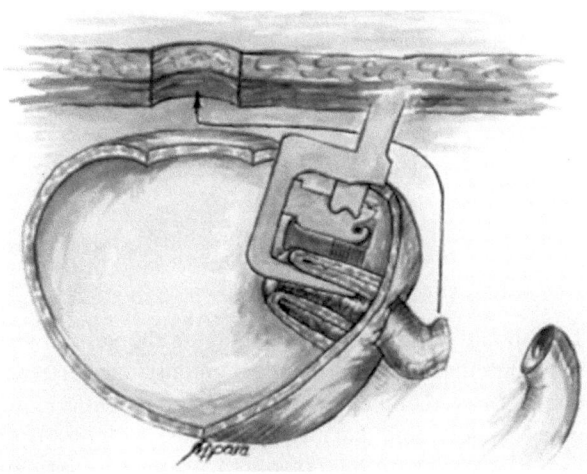

Fig. 17.5 Rotated pouch anchored to the bowel wall. New inlet sutured to the place for the former nipple valve

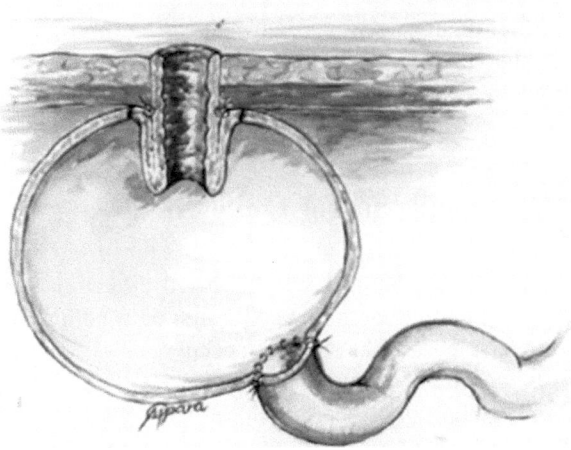

Fig. 17.6 New nipple
valve created by the use of
a more proximal bowel
segment

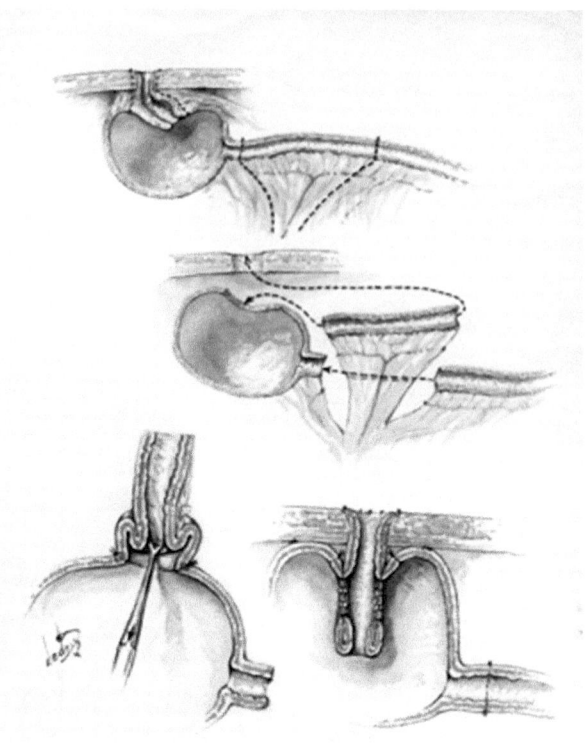

care should be taken to not damaging the vessels due to the fact that the isolated segment most often is dependent on only one set of marginal vessels. It is also crucial to assess that the new nipple valve and outlet is adequately circulated when the pouch is in its final position. The intussusception is probably easiest to make after the anastomosis of the transposed segment is completed. If the procedure is made without a separate pouch incision, the intussusception must be made after that about half the anastomosis is completed.

After the formal repair with some of the above methods, the pouch is attached to the abdominal wall in the conventional manner. A concomitant abdominal wall problem must of course be handled (see below).

17.9   Nipple and/or Outlet Stenosis

Conservative treatment with repeated dilatations, either with dilatators or endoscopic balloon dilatation, should first be tried and for a group of patients this will suffice, at least in the short perspective.

In the case of failure of the above strategies, laparotomy is necessary. A relatively short stricture in or near the tip of the nipple, could be managed with a local stricturotomy. After the stricture is cut, the edges should be sutured for hemostasis.

A promising alternative approach with endoscopic needle knife stricturotomy has been described in a case report by Shen et al.

In the case of longer strictures, the only option is one of the methods for nipple replacement described previously.

An isolated, deeper stricture to the outlet could, in principle, be treated with a new outlet made from a transposition of proximal bowel similar as for a transposition of the whole nipple outlet complex.

17.10 Abdominal Wall Problems

In our experience, it is quite common that the attachment of the pouch to the abdominal wall is the main problem. This is very often combined with a widening of the stomal passage through the fascia and some degree of slipping of the nipple valve.

Appropriate repair of the nipple is made as described above. If possible, a narrowing is made of the fascial opening with non-absorbable sutures, and if necessary combined with a sub-lay mesh. Sometimes the best option is to move the pouch to the other side of the abdomen, thus creating a new stoma.

The reason for loosening of the abdominal wall attachment for a small group of patients seems to be that they form very few or no adhesions. One solution in this situation could be the use of a mesh for optimizing the anchoring sutures. The mesh could also be exposed directly to the pouch for even better stability. One should be aware of the risk for developing fistulas when using a mesh.

17.11 Stomal Hernia

Even without slipping of the nipple, this condition can give problems with intubation. Repair is made as for nipple prolapse (see below), but without re-stapling if the nipple valve is fully competent. As an alternative, a local repair without laparotomy could be considered.

17.12 Fistula

Fistulas from the nipple base is certainly not that common as when mesh reinforcement of the nipple valve was thought to be part of the solution to nipple instability.

A local repair could be accomplished by excision of the fistula, preferably after partial des-invagination of the nipple, and a separate closure of the two bowel layers constituting the nipple valve.

When it is not feasible to make a repair in this manner, the nipple should be reconstructed, either with a rotation or as a transposed segment, as described above.

Fistulas from the pouch body are handled in the same way as for conventional enterocutaneous fistulas.

17.13   Strictures to the Inlet

Short strictures could be managed endoscopically with balloon dilatation. If the stricture is too long or if the dilatation fails it is easy to correct by a resection of the strictured segment and anastomosis.

17.14   Nipple Prolapse

A complete prolapse of the nipple through the stoma is rarely seen. The prolapse is most often easy to reduce manually, but will of course most likely recur. The condition is probably due to a too wide opening in the abdominal wall, and accordingly, a repair must include a reduction of that aperture. This is done with non-absorbable sutures, with or without a mesh. In the case of some degree of slipping, re-stapling and anchoring of the nipple to the pouch wall including strengthening of the nipple collar by a new row of sutures should be considered.

Local repair is described as an option. However, as it is often practically impossible to exclude nipple slipping without doing a complete examination, including detachment of the pouch from the abdominal wall, there is a risk of not solving the problem.

17.15   Superficial Stomal Strictures

As for strictures to the inlet or nipple, some superficial strictures of the stoma, could be dilated (mostly repeated) with some form of dilators, i.e. Hegar. Complementary local injections with steroids could be tried to soften the scar tissue.

However, most of these strictures must be corrected by excision of the stricture and dissection of the outlet down to the fascia, for enough length and minimizing of tension and re-suturing to the skin.

A bit more complex procedures, including a skin flap after partial excision of the full thickness scar, could also be used.

In some patients, though rare, the above strategies are not sufficient. It is in such cases possible to excise the entire outlet and replace it with a proximal segment in analogy with deeper outlet strictures.

17.16   Re-Do Repair

Even if revisional surgery is done under the most optimal conditions, recurrence unfortunately is not uncommon. Patients undergoing revision must be informed of the risk of failure and the subsequent need for additional surgery including pouch excision. Nevertheless, it is nearly always possible to make a secondary revision. Many of the patients are also asking for this. It is therefore in selected cases worth to proceed with both a second and third revision (or more) before giving up the pouch, as long as it is a fair chance to achieve a good function.

17.17 Resluts of Revisional Surgery

Several authors have reported on the frequency of revisional surgery and subsequent results, although differences in length of follow-up makes the interpretation of the data difficult.

Uniformly, problems with the nipple valve accounts for most of the revisional surgery, although the frequencies reported varies widely. There is also a clear trend to decreasing nipple problems with the refining of the technique of nipple construction combined with increasing experience. However, the issue of length of follow-up remains. In our experience, it is not that uncommon to see patients with a pouch that has functioned perfectly for more than 30 years, presenting with i.e. slipping of the nipple. Interestingly, it is not that uncommon that some of those patients has a history of pouch revision close in time to the primary construction.

Considering the results of revisional surgery, there is also the important issue of experience. The bulk of the literature is from the first decades after the initial reports and reflects the results of surgeons with a presumed experience that exceeds most of the surgeons active nowadays and definitely for what could be assumed for the coming generations. It is reasonable to believe that this fact will have a (negative) impact on the results of both primary and revisional surgery as the latter probably demands even more experience.

17.18 Conclusion

The Kock pouch is affected with an array of complications, particularly malfunctioning of the nipple valve. However, most of these are manageable with revisional surgery. Even after failed revisions, further re-revisions are worthwhile, with a reasonable prospect of regaining good pouch function.

Bibliography

1. Aytac E, et al. Is there still a role for continent ileostomy in the surgical treatment of inflammatory bowel disease? Inflamm Bowel Dis. 2014;20(12):2519–25.
2. Cranley B. The Kock reservoir ileostomy: a review of its development, problems and role in modern surgical practice. Br J Surg. 1983;70(2):94–9.
3. Denoya PI, et al. Delayed Kock pouch nipple valve failure: is revision indicated? Dis Colon Rectum. 2008;51(10):1544–7.

4. Dozois RR, et al. Improved results with continent ileostomy. Ann Surg. 1980;192(3):319–24.
5. Fazio VW, Church JM. Complications and function of the continent ileostomy at the Cleveland Clinic. World J Surg. 1988;12(2):148–54.
6. Goldman SL, Rombeau JL. The continent ileostomy: a collective review. Dis Colon Rectum. 1978;21(8):594–9.
7. Gottlieb LM, Handelsman JC. Treatment of outflow tract problems associated with continent ileostomy (Kock pouch). Report of six cases. Dis Colon Rectum. 1991;34(10):936–40.
8. Kann BR. Early stomal complications. Clin Colon Rectal Surg. 2008;21(1):23–30.
9. Keighley MRB. Keighley & Williams' surgery of the anus, rectum and colon. Boca Raton: CRC Press; 2018.
10. Kewenter and Brevinge in Rob & Smith's Operative surgery, Alimentary tract and abdominal wall.
11. Kock NG. Present status of the continent ileostomy: surgical revision of the malfunctioning ileostomy. Dis Colon Rectum. 1976;19(3):200–6.
12. Kock NG, et al. Ileostomy. Curr Probl Surg. 1977;14(8):1–52.
13. Lepisto AH, Jarvinen HJ. Durability of Kock continent ileostomy. Dis Colon Rectum. 2003;46(7):925–8.
14. Litle VR, et al. The continent ileostomy: long-term durability and patient satisfaction. J Gastrointest Surg. 1999;3(6):625–32.
15. Nessar G, et al. Long-term outcome and quality of life after continent ileostomy. Dis Colon Rectum. 2006;49(3):336–44.
16. Palmu A, Sivula A. Kock's continent ileostomy: results of 51 operations and experiences with correction of nipple-valve insufficiency. Br J Surg. 1978;65(9):645–8.
17. Parc Y, et al. The continent ileostomy: an alternative to end ileostomy? Short and long-term results of a single institution series. Dig Liver Dis. 2011;43(10):779–83.
18. Schrock TR. Complications of continent ileostomy. Am J Surg. 1979;138(1):162–9.
19. Chen M, Shen B. Endoscopic needle-knife stricturotomy for nipple valve stricture of continent ileostomy (with video). Gastrointest Endosc. 2015;81(5):1287–8. discussion 1288–1289.
20. Thompson JS, Williams SM. Technique for revision of continent ileostomy. Dis Colon Rectum. 1992;35(1):87–9.
21. Wasmuth HH, et al. Surgical load and long-term outcome for patients with Kock continent ileostomy. Color Dis. 2007;9(8):713–7.

Chapter 18
Failure

Hans H. Wasmuth and Mattias Block

18.1 Nipple Valve Slipping

The main cause of failure is nipple valve slipping. This phenomenon appears in 25–45% of the continent ileostomies. Most take place during the first 2–3 years, but can also appear later. The only treatment is surgical revision of the nipple.

There seem to be two main factors that jointly contribute to the process of nipple valve slipping. First, there is the entering of the mesentery into the nipple that creates a weakness in two ways. The base-suturing at this point has to be wider because sutures close to the mesentery can interfere with the blood supply to the nipple. The necessary adhesions formation will therefore not be optimal at the entering of the mesentery into the nipple. Further, the mass of the mesentery can contribute to loss of adhesions and therefore separate the two layers of the nipple. This process makes the area in the nipple and the entering open for forces acting on de-sussusception, hence the slipping.

Second, there is the loosing of the pouch attachment to the abdominal wall. The process of small bowel dettachment from the abdominal wall is a common process after all abdominal surgery. Adhesions become looser in the first year after surgery. Further, the intubation is not without resistant to the entering. The intubation manoeuvre is a force that will cause distress on the attachment. If there are any angulations or strictures, the increased force of intubation will but stress

H. H. Wasmuth
Department of Surgery, Colorectal Unit, St. Olavs Hospital, Trondheim University Hospital, Trondheim, Norway
e-mail: Hans.Wasmuth@stolav.no

M. Block (✉)
Department of Surgery, Sahlgrenska University Hospital, University of Gothenburg, Gothenburg, Sweden
e-mail: mattias.block@vgregion.se

© Springer Nature Switzerland AG 2019
P. Myrelid, M. Block (eds.), *The Kock Pouch*,
https://doi.org/10.1007/978-3-319-95591-9_18

on the anchoring of the pouch and so forth, the attachment to the abdominal wall. The anchoring will be softened and the attachment will not have any counter-force to the slipping.

When both these factors appear they will have synergetic effects. The force on the intussusception at the entering of the mesentery will pull the mesentery out of the nipple. The sutures of the nipple base will then gradually separate and the slipping-process starts. The process is maintained by intubation.

This result in nipple shortening which causes leakage to appear. The shortening is mainly affected at the mesentery site of the nipple. This is seen as a partial nipple slipping, nearly complete at the mesentery side and less so at the anti-mesentery side. The process can in some cases be more circumferential.

There are also other conditions that might trigger the slipping. The process of distention of the pouch after 2 weeks past construction can affect the sutures at the base of the nipple as well and the anchoring sutures. In the long run the filling and emptying of the pouch is dynamic. This dynamic movement has to end with an equilibrium that do not destabilize the base and the position of the pouch. Otherwise the slipping might be enhanced.

The peristaltic movement of the bowel in the nipple is not coordinated to be in a stable intussusception mode. The peristalsis might act more on the de-sussusception tendency.

The stabilisation of the nipple is dependent on the formation of tight adhesions. The sutures and staplers are there to facilitate the creation of the adhesions. Without the adhesions, formation of the nipple will eventually fail. It is therefore not advisable to offer continent ileostomy to patients with deficiency in the collagen structure, such as patients with Ehler-Danlos syndrome.

18.2   Nipple Prolapse

The nipple prolapse is not common and is only reported sporadically in the literature. This complication appears suddenly at the moment when the whole nipple or parts of the nipple everts and become externalised above skin level. This protrusion is not continent. The blood supply can also be disturbed.

The process has its origin in the hole of the abdominal wall where the stoma segment of the nipple enters. The diameter of this opening can be wide enough for allowing the pouch-wall to bulge into the abdominal wall. The abdominal pressure may then act in this small hernia at the base of the nipple to start an eversion of the nipple. The distention of the continent pouch will facilitate the eversion process in a rapid way.

This phenomenon has been observed in pregnancy and after revisional surgery when the opening in the abdominal wall has been widened through surgical trauma when taking down the stoma.

18.3   Other Reasons for Failure

18.3.1   Multiple Revisional Surgical Procedures

Patients with a functioning Kock pouch have a very good quality of life and are extremely satisfied with their pouch. However, if the pouch become malfunctioning and requiries revisional surgery, there is an upper limit of how many procedures the patient (and the surgeon) can manage. If multiple revisions have been performed and there are still some problems with the pouch, discussion with the patient of excising the pouch and create an end-ileostomy should be initiated. There is no upper limit of surgical procedures being performed, it is always a decision that the patient and the surgeon make together. Different centres have reported as much as up to 15–17 revisional procedures, although not all of these have been laparotomies, ie some re-operations have "only" consist of skin- and/or subcutaneous procedures. But again, the final decision is up to the patient and the surgeon.

18.3.2   Mental Instability

Being one of the contraindications, mental instability is an important factor to consider before making a Kock pouch. Even though the patient can be mentally prepared and motivated before the primary construction of the pouch, hesitations can arise along the road and there have been occasions when Kock pouches have been removed to patient preferences even if the pouch is functionally intact and stable.

18.3.3   Patient Preference

See above.

18.3.4   Crohn's disease

As described in one of the previous chapters, patients with Crohn's disease have a higher risk of complications and failure than other patients. Some authors report a failure-rate as high as 60% and 70% after 10 and 20 years, respectively.

18.3.5 Pouchitis

Chapter 12 has discussed pouchitis in details. If the pouchitis turns out to be chronic with frequent emptying of the pouch, abdominal pain, fever and a feeling of sickness, and if the chronic pouchitis in addition turns out to be resistant to medical therapy and/or intubation of the pouch, failure is at risk. However, as with chronic pouchitis in pelvic pouches, chronic pouchitis is a rare cause of failure in the Kock pouch.

18.3.6 Dysplasia and/or Cancer

Dysplasia is uncommon in the Kock pouch and cancer even more so. It should be stressed that cancer in the Kock pouch is extremely unusual. In the literature there has only been one official report. High-grade dysplasia and cancer are of course indications for pouch removal, similar to the situation regarding pelvic pouches. Low-grade dysplasia is different and pouch removal is not mandatory. Most authors recommend endoscopic evaluation with multiple biopsies every 6 months in the presence of low-grade dysplasia.

Bibliography

1. Behrens DT, et al. Conversion of failed ileal pouch-anal anastomosis to continent ileostomy. Dis Colon Rectum. 1999;42(4):490–5. discussion 495-496.
2. Börjesson L, et al. The failed pelvic pouch: conversion to a continent ileostomy. Tech Coloproctol. 2004a;8(2):102–5.
3. Börjesson L, et al. The failed pelvic pouch: conversion to a continent ileostomy. Tech Coloproctol. 2004b;8(2):102–5.
4. Hultén L, et al. The failing pelvic pouch conversion to continent ileostomy. Int J Color Dis. 1992;7(3):119–21.
5. Wasmuth HH, et al. Failed pelvic pouch substituted by continent ileostomy. Color Dis. 2010;12(7 Online):e109–13.
6. Goldman SL, Rombeau JL. The continent ileostomy: a collective review. Dis Colon Rectum. 1978;21(8):594–9.
7. Lepistö AH, Järvinen HJ. Durability of Kock continent ileostomy. Dis Colon Rectum. 2003;46(7):925–8.
8. Litle VR, et al. The continent ileostomy: long-term durability and patient satisfaction. J Gastrointest Surg. 1999;3(6):625–32.
9. Nessar G, et al. Long-term outcome and quality of life after continent ileostomy. Dis Colon Rectum. 2006;49(3):336–44.
10. Wasmuth HH, et al. Surgical load and long-term outcome for patients with Kock continent ileostomy. Color Dis. 2007;9(8):713–7.
11. Beck DE. Clinical aspects of continent ileostomies. Clin Colon Rectal Surg. 2004;17(1):57–63.
12. Castillo E, et al. Continent ileostomy: current experience. Dis Colon Rectum. 2005;48(6):1263–8.

13. Nessar G, Wu JS. Evolution of continent ileostomy. World J Gastroenterol. 2012;18(27):3479–82.

14. Hashavia E, et al. Risk factors for chronic pouchitis after ileal pouch-anal anastomosis: a prospective cohort study. Color Dis. 2012;14(11):1365–71.

15. Landy J, et al. Etiology of pouchitis. Inflamm Bowel Dis. 2012;18(6):1146–55.

16. Um JW, M'Koma AE. Pouch-related dysplasia and adenocarcinoma following restorative proctocolectomy for ulcerative colitis. Tech Coloproctol. 2011;15(1):7–16.

17. Thompson-Fawcett MW, et al. Risk of dysplasia in long-term ileal pouches and pouches with chronic pouchitis. Gastroenterology. 2001;121(2):275–81.

18. Chen KK, et al. Histopathological changes in Kock pouch. Br J Urol. 1993;72(4):433–40.

19. Cox CL, et al. Development of invasive adenocarcinoma in a long-standing Kock continent ileostomy: report of a case. Dis Colon Rectum. 1997;40(4):500–3.

Chapter 19
Alternative Methods to the Kock Continent Ileostomy

Tom Øresland

19.1 Introduction

The Kock pouch although a great innovation and a huge improvement in quality of life at the time it was introduced never gained worldwide acceptance. Many were those who came to Gothenburg to "see one, do one, and maybe teach one", of course this was doomed to fail. The procedure is not only complicated in that it includes several intricate steps but also the postoperative care is probably crucial for a successful outcome and this was seldom recognized. Due to this the procedure got a not so well deserved reputation of being burdened by complications and all sorts of difficulties. However, these circumstances lead some surgeons to design alternatives striving of hopefully finding an improved continent pouch. The most well-known are the Barnett Continent Ileostomy Reservoir and the T- pouch, both emanating from the United States. Their acceptance has been even less than that for the originator, but still at least the Barnett reservoir is used to some extent. Then there are a couple of alternative methods that have been tried but so far none of them has been launched into clinical practice.

19.2 The Barnett Continent Ileostomy Reservoir

The Barnett continent ileostomy was first described in its first version in 1982 and it was gradually refined over the next years. There have been few publications on the procedure; by large it seems to perform as the Kock pouch both in achieving continence and being burdened by reoperations. The last published report from 1995 was

T. Øresland (✉)
Clinic for Surgical Sciences, University of Oslo and Department of Gi Surgery, Akeshus University Hospital, Oslo, Norway
e-mail: tom.oresland@medisin.uio.no

© Springer Nature Switzerland AG 2019
P. Myrelid, M. Block (eds.), *The Kock Pouch*,
https://doi.org/10.1007/978-3-319-95591-9_19

a multicenter report from five US clinics with altogether 510 patients and a mean follow up just above 2 years. The publication is quite optimistic, a network with a registry and future reports are spoken of but then nothing is published. The actual results seem as good as could be expected for the Kock pouch. They reported a pouch excision rate of 6.5%, major repairs in 13% and all over pouch related re-operative surgery in 21% of the patients. The majority of patients intubated the pouch 3–5 times daily and the majority also reported good to excellent quality of life with 22% reporting excessive mucous secretions (see below). For the time being there seems to be one active center in California that is devoted to only the Barnett pouch, there is also a quite active face book group and you can read fancy advertisements on the internet.

The construction of this pouch includes a collar of small bowel encircling the distal part of the nipple valve adding to its stability. At the time this was invented a synthetic mesh was used as a collar to stabilize the nipple valve, however just like in the Kock pouch this was abandoned due to mesh migration and fistula formation. The "living collar" is supposedly doing the same job but without the risks. The pouch is made out of approximately 60–65 cm of the terminal ileum (45 cm for a Kock pouch) and the segment used for the pouch is divided from the oral ileum (Fig. 19.1). The continence valve is made mainly in the same as in the Kock pouch with an intussusception stabilized by three stapler rows, the difference being that it is made on an iso-peristaltic bowel segment. This would allow the mucous to be

Fig. 19.1 The terminal ileum is divided 60–65 cm from its end. The oral part will be used for the pouch outlet and the continence valve, the middle part will form the pouch and the aboral part will form the "living collar" that stabilizes the continence valve

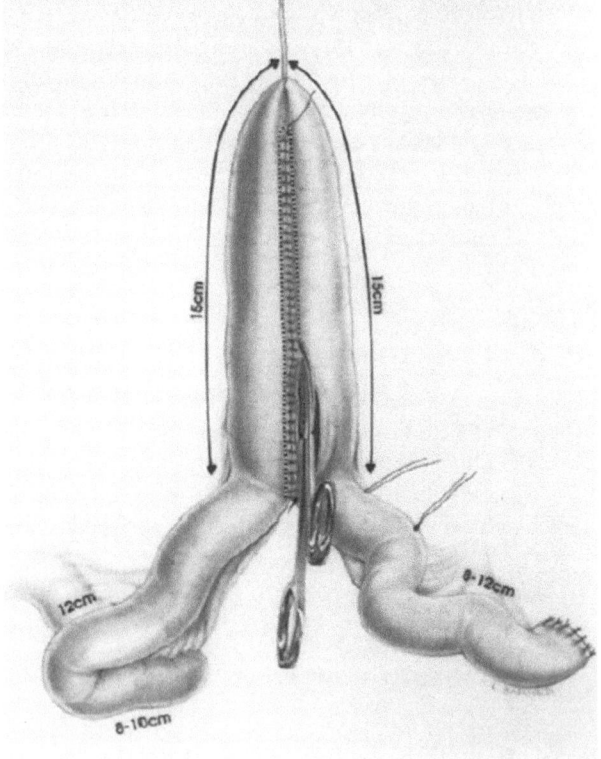

drained into the pouch rather than out outwards into the stoma. In the Kock pouch the nipple valve is constructed on the end of the bowel and is primarily anti-peristaltic which is pointed to as a disadvantage. Neither is the pouch double folded, but folded longitudinally as a J-pouch. This was to avoid the trifurcated suture line that is included in the Kock pouch construction which could be a potential risk for leaks in the newly constructed pouch. The construction seems at least as complicated as that for the Kock pouch. The advantage of these differences seems mostly theoretical. Leaks from the suture lines of the pouch are extremely seldom seen in the newly constructed Kock pouch, they are reported in the Barnett pouch. When re-operating on Kock pouches for nipple valve dysfunction a common method is to make a new valve on the inlet side of the pouch dividing the bowel 15 cm oral to the inlet and using this segment for a new iso-peristaltic valve, however no definite advantages of this have been proven.

19.2.1 Construction of the Barnett Continent Reservoir (Figs. 19.2, 19.3, 19.4 and 19.5)

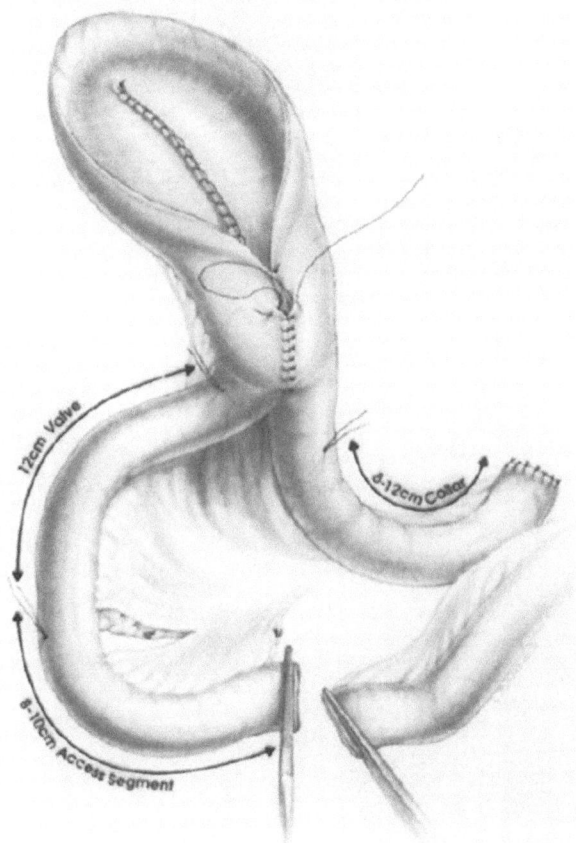

Fig. 19.2 A J-pouch is formed of the middle segment

Fig. 19.3 The bowel is
intussuscepted and secured
with staplers to form the
nipple valve

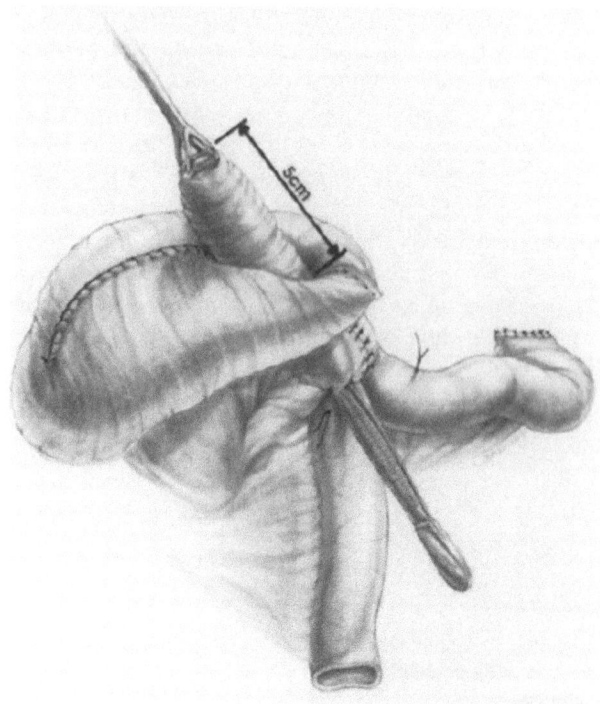

Fig. 19.4 The closed
aboral end is drawn
through a hole in the
mesentery to form a sling
around the pouch outlet,
the "living collar"

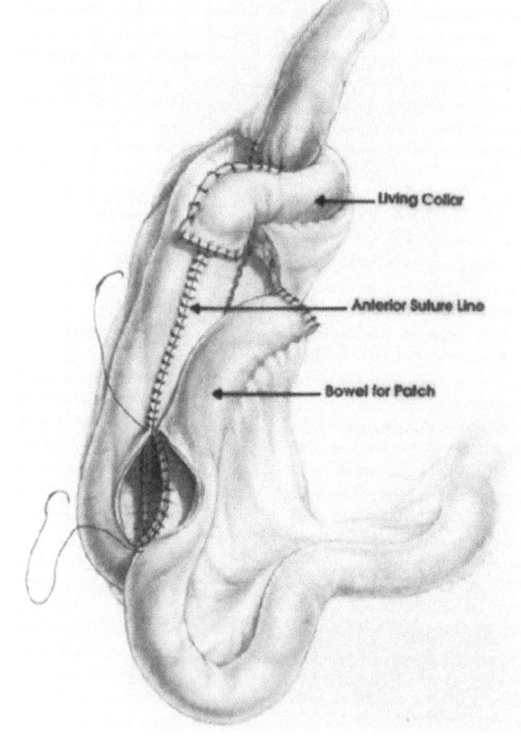

Fig. 19.5 The oral bowel is sutured side to side into the J- pouch to complete the construction which is the attached to the inside of the abdominal wall on the predetermined stoma site

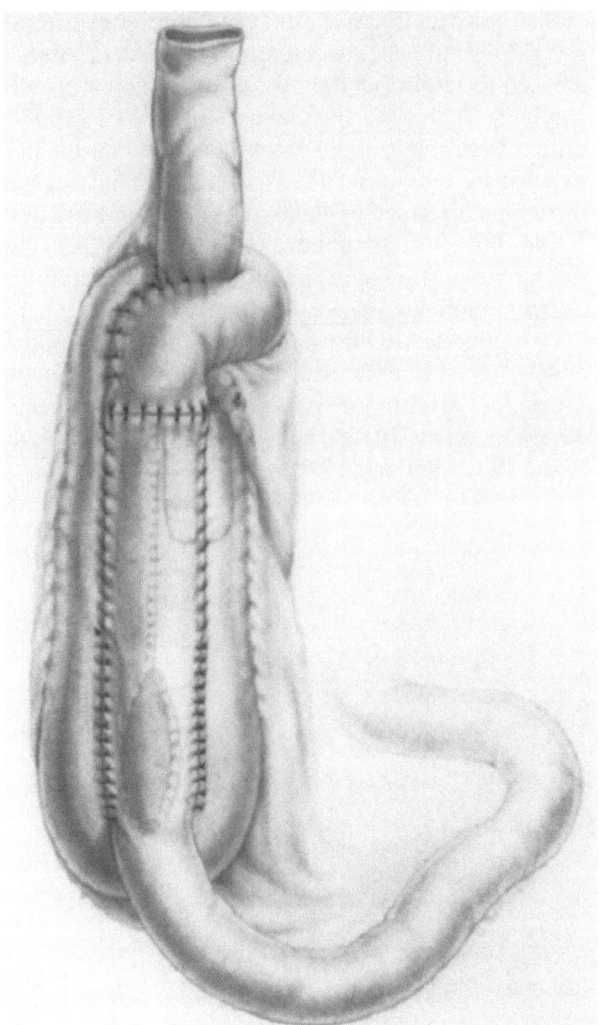

19.3 The T-Pouch

The T-pouch was described by Stein in 1999 and then by Kaiser, the last publication is from 2012 giving a collective experience over 10 years with 40 patients. Median follow-up was 6.2 years. There were some immediate complications with five anastomotic leaks, five fistulas and one valve necrosis and some other minor complications. Patients intubated on average four times a day and the 36 patients that still were having their T-pouches were by large continent. Mucous seepage and dietary restrictions were experienced. The authors did not seem overly enthusiastic and the report is hampered by a long inclusion time, relatively few patients and a short follow-up.

The construction was first used in urology after that the urologist had started using Kock pouches to create neo-bladders after radical cystectomies. It was devised to minimize the all too well-known problems with the intussuscepted continence valve mechanism used in the Kock and Barnett pouches. The T-pouch differs from the original Kock pouch in that the continence mechanism is constructed by encircling the isolated terminal segment of the ileum in a serosa lined tunnel formed by the two apposed limbs of bowel that will form the pouch. A non-intussuscepting valve is thus formed in an attempt to further diminish the risk of valve slippage. The drawings and descriptions give the impression of a rather complicated procedure and it should probably not be attempted without having good instructions and training from a colleague familiar with the procedure. This of course also applies to the Barnett pouch. The literature on the T-pouch is even more sparse and nothing has been heard of it in the scientific databases since 2012 when the first 10 years with 40 patients were reported (Figs. 19.6, 19.7 and 19.8).

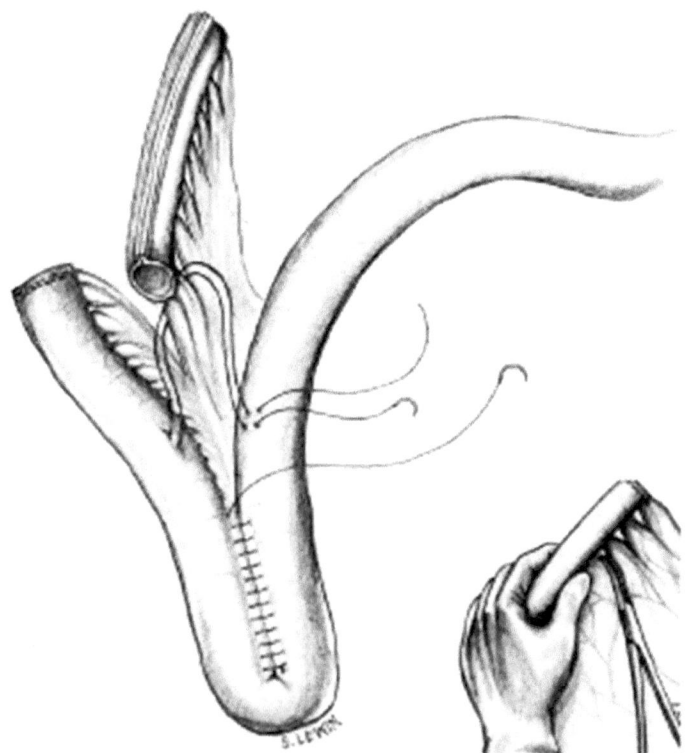

Fig. 19.6 The isolated terminal ileum is stapled along its anti-mesenteric side to make the diameter fit snugly around an emptying catheter. This segment is the sutures to the serosa of the two 20 cm limbs that will form the pouch

Fig. 19.7 The pouch limbs are opened up with two wider flaps at the level of the outlet segment. These flaps are then sutured over the outlet encircling it

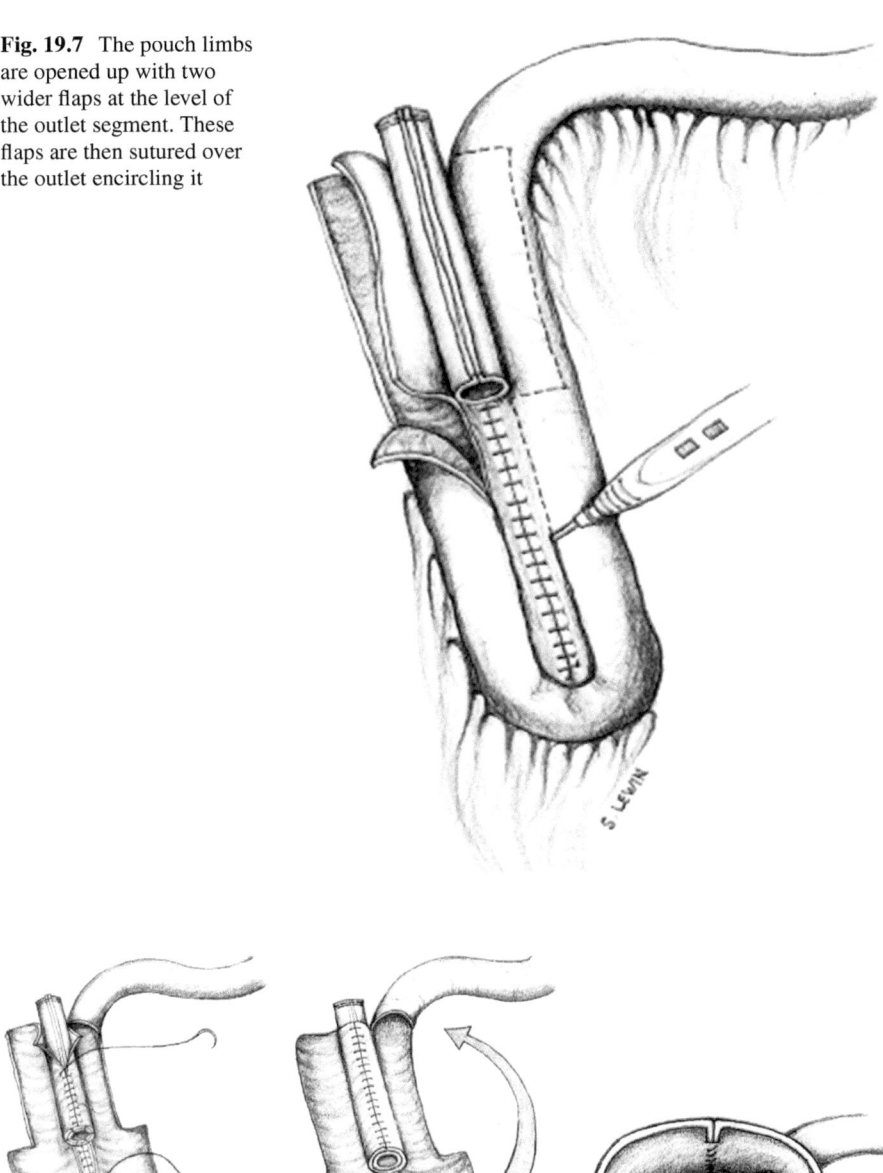

Fig. 19.8 The back wall of the pouch is sutured up to the valve. The pouch is then folded transversely and sutured according to the principles of the Kock pouch. The protruding outlet segment is drawn through the abdominal wall to form the stoma

19.4   Occlusion Devices

19.4.1   Intraluminal Balloon Occlusion

John Pemberton in 1984 published on occluding the ileostomy with an indwelling balloon catheter. Progressive stoma occlusion with an indwelling occluding device was evaluated in four healthy patients with Brooke end-ileostomies. Eventually occlusion periods of 5–8 h were reached and it seemed that developed a pre-stoma reservoir after 10–16 weeks. No negative effects on absorption of glucose, electrolytes, vitamin B12 and fat could be noted. The appearance of the mucosa did not change as evaluated on endoscopy. Although it was stated that patients achieved reliable continence the project does not seem to have been taken further into clinical practice.

19.4.2   Magnetic Stoma Cap

In the late 1970s the magnetic occlusion device was used in several studies emanating from Erlangen in Germany, trying to achieve a continent colostomy. A rather ingenious thought with two magnets, one circular embedded in the subcutaneous fat surrounding the stoma and the other shaped as a lid with a central tap containing the other magnet pole introduced into the stoma. The magnetic forces would then keep the lid in an exact position occluding the stoma opening without excreting any pressure on the bowel wall leading up to the stoma opening. The occlusion was also achieved by the cap exerting some pressure on the skin surrounding the stoma. The device was tried first in animals and ten at several centers in patients but it never became universally available and to the author's knowledge it is no longer in use. It was originally designed for colostomies and never reported tried in ileostomies. However from Australia it is now reported on a revival of this old idea in a more sophisticated form intended both for colostomies and ileostomies. The company can be found on the internet (Stomalife) but so far there are no good indications reported or whether it will work in practice or not (Figs. 19.9 and 19.10).

19.4.3   TIES

The TIES (Transcutaneous Implant Evacuation System) device is a more recent innovation consisting of a titanium ring with a solid outer part and a mesh extension into the subcuticular tissue. The ileum is brought through this ring and will grow into the titanium beaded surface. After a healing period a lid can be applied to the solid outer part. The TIES device has been developed over several years starting with animal experiments and then it has been tested on patients in two different versions. A handful of patients has this far been operated with first one version and then

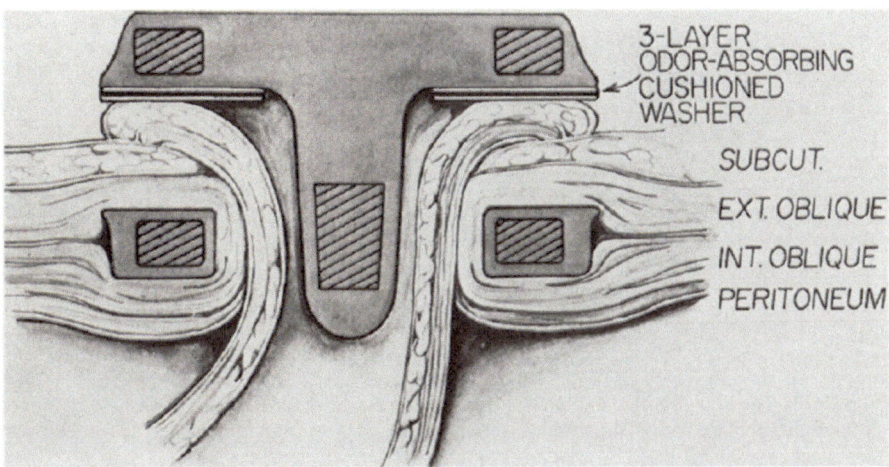

Fig. 19.9 The original magnetic occlusion device

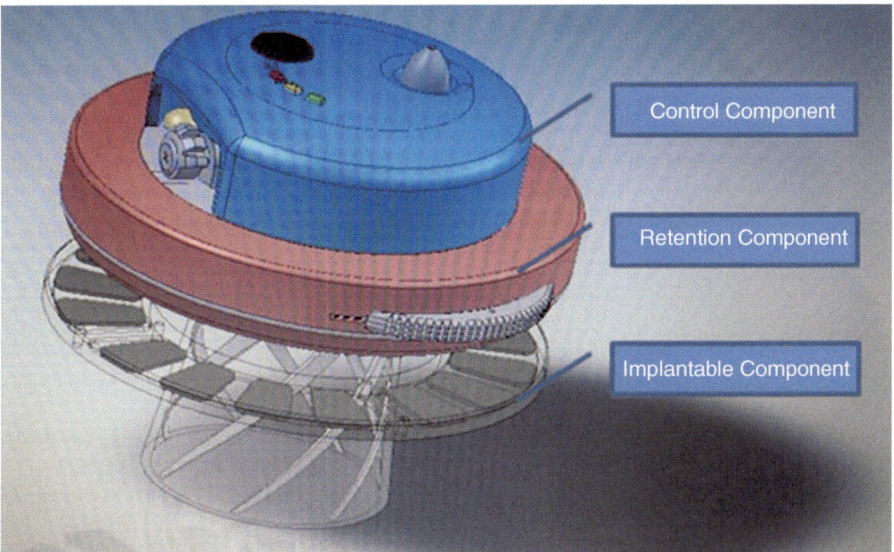

Fig. 19.10 The new "Stomalife" stoma occlusion device

a further developed version of the titanium ring. There were surprisingly few serious adverse advents related to the device itself but for both the versions the problem is the exact ingrowth. The main problem is that the bowel does not attach itself to the protruding solid part of the titanium device thus continence is seldom achieved. For the time being the future of the TIES system seems very uncertain and if not further developed it will probably fail to work as intended (the author's personal experience) (Fig. 19.11).

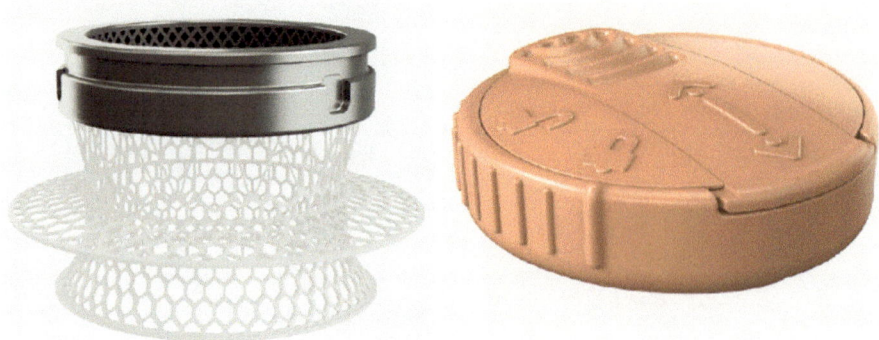

Fig. 19.11 The titanium implant, the solid part protrudes above the skin level. The bowel is drawn through the implant and is supposed to attach all the way up to the top of the solid outer part. Continence is then achieved by applying the lid

19.5   Summary

The alternatives to the original Kock continent ileostomy described above do not seem to be better than the originator, only the Barnett continent ileostomy reservoir is still in use and offers a comparable outcome. Having to live with an incontinent stoma is problematic in many aspects of life and the quest for better solutions than those we have today will hopefully continue. The demand for a well working continent ileostomy that is reliable and that can be constructed by the average colorectal surgeon is still prevailing and hopefully we will see new solutions in the future.

Bibliography

1. Barnett WO. Continent Ileostomy. South Med J. 1983;76(5):583–6.
2. Mullen P, Behrens D, Chalmers T, et al. Barnett continent intestinal reservoir. Multicenter experience with an alternative to the Brooke ileostomy. Dis Colon Rectum. 1995;38(6):573–82.
3. Stein JP, Buscarini M, De Filippo RE, Skinner DG. Application of the T pouch as an ileo-anal reservoir. J Urol. 1999;162(6):2052–3.
4. Kaiser AM, Stein JP, Beart RW Jr. T-pouch: a new valve design for a continent ileostomy. Dis Colon Rectum. 2002;45(3):411–5.
5. Kaiser AM. T-pouch: results of the first 10 years with a nonintussuscepting continent ileostomy. Dis Colon Rectum. 2012;55(2):155–62.
6. Stein JP, Lieskovsky G, Ginsberg DA, Bochner BH, Skinner DG. The T pouch: an orthotopic ileal neobladder incorporating a serosal lined ileal antireflux technique. J Urol. 1998;159(6):1836–42.
7. Pemberton JH, van Heerden JA, Beart RW Jr, Kelly KA, Phillips SF, Taylor BM. A continent ileostomy device. Ann Surg. 1983;197(5):618–26.
8. Feustel H, Hennig G, Filler D, Hubner E. Continent colostomy through magnetic closure in animal experiments on dogs. Langenbecks Arch Chir. 1975;(Suppl):337–40.
9. Bauer JJ, Wertkin MG, Gelernt IM, Kreel I. A continent colostomy: the magnetic stoma cap. Am J Surg. Sep 1977;134(3):334–7.

10. Feustel H, Hennig G. Colostomy continence achieved with an implanted circular magnet (author's transl). Dtsch Med Wochenschr. 1975;100(19):1063–4.
11. Husemann B, Hager T. Experience with the Erlangen magnetic ring colostomy-closure system. Int Surg. 1984;69(4):297–300.
12. Kewenter J. Continent colostomy with the aid of a magnetic closing system: a preliminary report. Dis Colon Rectum. 1978;21(1):46–51.
13. Bauer JJ. The magnetic stoma cap: a continent colostomy current status. Curr Surg. 1983;40(1):1–3.
14. Strigard K, Oresland T, Rutegard J, Gunnarsson U. Transcutaneous implant evacuation system: a new approach to continent stoma construction. Color Dis. 2011;13(11):e379–82.

Index

© Springer Nature Switzerland AG 2019
P. Myrelid, M. Block (eds.), *The Kock Pouch*,
https://doi.org/10.1007/978-3-319-95591-9